# HELP YOUR DOG
# FIGHT
# CANCER

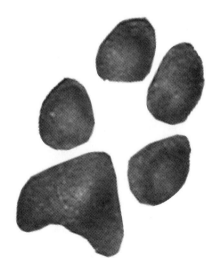

# HELP YOUR DOG FIGHT CANCER

## WHAT EVERY CARETAKER SHOULD KNOW

## ABOUT CANINE CANCER

FEATURING BULLET'S SURVIVAL STORY

by Laurie Kaplan, MSC

Founder and administrator of The Magic Bullet Fund

The information in this book applies to canines. Some therapies, treatments and methods discussed in this book may be harmful if applied to other species of animals with or without cancer.

Great care has been taken to ensure the accuracy of the information presented in good conscience herein and to ensure that no methods are described that could be harmful to your dog. However, the author and publisher make no warranty, express or implied, regarding the efficacy of treatments or home care techniques discussed in this book and are not to be held liable for consequences from the application of those treatments or techniques. The author and publisher have done everything reasonably possible to ensure that this book is accurate and up-to-date. Veterinary oncology is a dynamic and ever changing field. Cancer treatments evolve, new information becomes available and recommended treatments and procedures are constantly revised. Some advice and strategies discussed in this book may not be suitable for your particular situation. The anatomy, condition, age, medical history and particulars of any canine are unique and not all recommendations are appropriate for every dog. This book is not intended as veterinary medical advice nor to supplant appropriate veterinary medical consultation. Readers are advised to always consult with a veterinarian.

*Forgive the assignment of masculine pronouns to both humans and canines in this book. This does not reflect sexism, it reflects only a desire not to liter the text content of this book with "he/she"s.*

2nd Edition
Printed in the U.S.A.
Publisher JanGen Press, Briarcliff NY, 2008
Copyright © 2008 Laurie Kaplan, all rights reserved.
Library of Congress Control Number: 2008923705
ISBN: 978097547947-6

1st Edition
Printed in the U.S.A.
Publisher JanGen Press, Briarcliff NY, 2004
Copyright © 2004 Laurie Kaplan, all rights reserved.
2nd Printing March, 2005
Library of Congress Control Number: 2004107152
ISBN: 0-9754794-6-6

*Cover photograph by Tracy M. Basile*
*Cover design by Kim Leonard/Bookcovers.com*

*This book is dedicated to Bullet, my brave little boy*
*the love of my life*
*the dog of my dreams*

*and*

*To all of the Brave Spirits who will fight*
*for another shining moment in the loving arms*
*of their special person.*

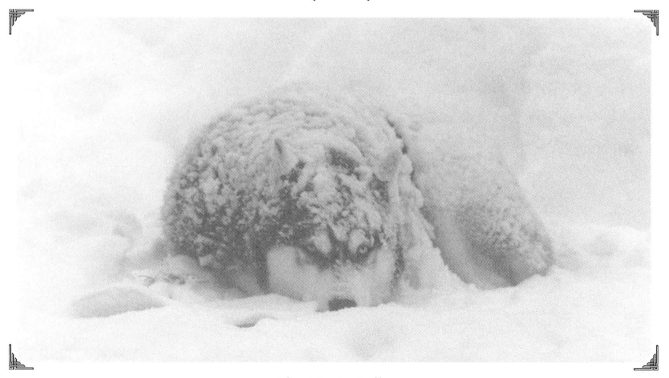

*The Magic Bullet*
*March 15, 1991 ~ November 20, 2004*

# CONTENTS

Introduction . . . . . . . . . . . . . . . . . . . . . . . . . . . . . . . . . . . . . . . . . . . . . . . . . . . . i

Author's Foreword. . . . . . . . . . . . . . . . . . . . . . . . . . . . . . . . . . . . . . . . . . . . . . iii

**Bullet's Story, Part One: Prologue** . . . . . . . . . . . . . . . . . . . . . . . . . . . . . . . . .1

| | | | |
|---|---|---|---|
| CHAPTER | 1 | **Prepare For Battle** . . . . . . . . . . . . . . . . . . . . . . . . . . . . . . . . . . . . . **9** |

Not Today . . . . . . . . . . . . . . . . . . . . . . . . . . . . . . . . . . . . . . . . . . . .10

Keep A Log . . . . . . . . . . . . . . . . . . . . . . . . . . . . . . . . . . . . . . . . . . .11

Don't Be Afraid To Ask . . . . . . . . . . . . . . . . . . . . . . . . . . . . . . . . . .12

Sidebar: No Contract . . . . . . . . . . . . . . . . . . . . . . . . . . . . .12

Illustration: Lymph Node Locations . . . . . . . . . . . . . . . . . .13

Sidebar: Resources on the Net . . . . . . . . . . . . . . . . . . . . . .15

Read, Read, Read . . . . . . . . . . . . . . . . . . . . . . . . . . . . . . . . . . . . . .16

"It's Just A Dog!" . . . . . . . . . . . . . . . . . . . . . . . . . . . . . . . . . . . . . . .16

CHAPTER   2   **Early Decisions**. . . . . . . . . . . . . . . . . . . . . . . . . . . . . . . . . . . . . . . . **19**

Sidebar: Decisions You Can Make . . . . . . . . . . . . . . . . . . . .20

Treatment Decisions . . . . . . . . . . . . . . . . . . . . . . . . . . . . . . . . . . .21

Choosing A Doctor . . . . . . . . . . . . . . . . . . . . . . . . . . . . . . . . . . . .22

Sidebar: Assemble Your Team . . . . . . . . . . . . . . . . . . . . . . .23

Schools of Veterinary Medicine . . . . . . . . . . . . . . . . . . . . . . . . . .25

To Test or Not To Test . . . . . . . . . . . . . . . . . . . . . . . . . . . . . . . . . .26

To Treat or Not to Treat . . . . . . . . . . . . . . . . . . . . . . . . . . . . . . . .27

Financial Considerations . . . . . . . . . . . . . . . . . . . . . . . . . . . . . . .27

Sidebar: Considerations for Treatment . . . . . . . . . . . . . . . .28

Get a Move On! . . . . . . . . . . . . . . . . . . . . . . . . . . . . . . . . . . . . . .29

CHAPTER   3   **About Canine Cancer** . . . . . . . . . . . . . . . . . . . . . . . . . . . . . . . . . . **31**

Types of Canine Cancer . . . . . . . . . . . . . . . . . . . . . . . . . . . . . . . .32

Sidebar: The Most Common Canine Cancers . . . . . . . . . . . .33

Why Dogs Get Cancer . . . . . . . . . . . . . . . . . . . . . . . . . . . . . . . . .34

CHAPTER   4   **Medical Interventions** . . . . . . . . . . . . . . . . . . . . . . . . . . . . . . . . . **39**

Diagnostics . . . . . . . . . . . . . . . . . . . . . . . . . . . . . . . . . . . . . . . . . .39

Surgical Interventions . . . . . . . . . . . . . . . . . . . . . . . . . . . . . . . . . .40

*Knowledge Is Power, by Dr. Philip J. Bergman* . . . . . . . . . . . .*42*

Radiation Therapy . . . . . . . . . . . . . . . . . . . . . . . . . . . . . . . . . . . .43

Therapies in the Pipeline . . . . . . . . . . . . . . . . . . . . . . . . . . . . . . .44

Clinical Trials . . . . . . . . . . . . . . . . . . . . . . . . . . . . . . . . . . . . . . . .48

Comparative Oncology . . . . . . . . . . . . . . . . . . . . . . . . . . . . . . . .49

Early Detection . . . . . . . . . . . . . . . . . . . . . . . . . . . . . . . . . . . . . .50

CHAPTER  5     **Chemotherapy** . . . . . . . . . . . . . . . . . . . . . . . . . . . . . . . . . . . . . . . . . . . . . **53**
                *Early Detection of Cancer or of Relapse, by Dr. Rodney Page* . . . . . . . . . . . . . . . . . *54*
                Chemotherapy Simplified . . . . . . . . . . . . . . . . . . . . . . . . . . . . . . . . . . . . . . . . .56
                    Sidebar: About Protocols . . . . . . . . . . . . . . . . . . . . . . . . . . . . . . . . . . . . . .57
                Chemotherapy Agents . . . . . . . . . . . . . . . . . . . . . . . . . . . . . . . . . . . . . . . . . .58
                A Delicate Procedure . . . . . . . . . . . . . . . . . . . . . . . . . . . . . . . . . . . . . . . . . . .59
                Chemotherapy Leaks . . . . . . . . . . . . . . . . . . . . . . . . . . . . . . . . . . . . . . . . . . .60
                Bullet's Chemo Experience . . . . . . . . . . . . . . . . . . . . . . . . . . . . . . . . . . . . . . .61

CHAPTER  6     **Side Effects** . . . . . . . . . . . . . . . . . . . . . . . . . . . . . . . . . . . . . . . . . . . . . . . . **63**
                *Keep Your Dog Healthy During Chemotherapy, by Dr. Kevin A. Hahn* . . . . . . . . . *64*
                Don't Panic! . . . . . . . . . . . . . . . . . . . . . . . . . . . . . . . . . . . . . . . . . . . . . . . . .68
                Bullet's Side Effects . . . . . . . . . . . . . . . . . . . . . . . . . . . . . . . . . . . . . . . . . . .72
                    Sidebar: Chemotherapy Agents and Side Effects  . . . . . . . . . . . . . . . . . . . . .70

CHAPTER  7     **What's For Dinner?** . . . . . . . . . . . . . . . . . . . . . . . . . . . . . . . . . . . . . . . . . **75**
                Feeding Naturally . . . . . . . . . . . . . . . . . . . . . . . . . . . . . . . . . . . . . . . . . . . . .76
*COLOR PLATE         Bullet's Cancer Diet, Illustrated  . . . . . . . . . . . . . . . . . . . . . . . . . . . . .C1-C4
                    Special Offers for your dog  . . . . . . . . . . . . . . . . . . . . . . . . . . . . . . . .C5-C8
                Is A Raw Diet Safe? . . . . . . . . . . . . . . . . . . . . . . . . . . . . . . . . . . . . . . . . . . .77
                How Hard Can It Be? . . . . . . . . . . . . . . . . . . . . . . . . . . . . . . . . . . . . . . . . . .78
                Bullet's Pre-Cancer Diet . . . . . . . . . . . . . . . . . . . . . . . . . . . . . . . . . . . . . . . .79
                    Sidebar: Bullet's Cancer Diet Ingredients . . . . . . . . . . . . . . . . . . . . . . . . .79
                About Bullet's Cancer Diet . . . . . . . . . . . . . . . . . . . . . . . . . . . . . . . . . . . . . .80
                Water . . . . . . . . . . . . . . . . . . . . . . . . . . . . . . . . . . . . . . . . . . . . . . . . . . . . .81
                Feeding Frozen . . . . . . . . . . . . . . . . . . . . . . . . . . . . . . . . . . . . . . . . . . . . . .82
                    Sidebar: Leading a Dog to...Meat-Jello! . . . . . . . . . . . . . . . . . . . . . . . . . .81
                Variety for Life . . . . . . . . . . . . . . . . . . . . . . . . . . . . . . . . . . . . . . . . . . . . . .83
                Don't Forget the Treats! . . . . . . . . . . . . . . . . . . . . . . . . . . . . . . . . . . . . . . . .84

CHAPTER  8     **What Else Can I Do?** . . . . . . . . . . . . . . . . . . . . . . . . . . . . . . . . . . . . . . . . **87**
                To Supplement or Not . . . . . . . . . . . . . . . . . . . . . . . . . . . . . . . . . . . . . . . . . .88
                    Sidebar: Decisions You Can Make  . . . . . . . . . . . . . . . . . . . . . . . . . . . . . .89
                Slow Down . . . . . . . . . . . . . . . . . . . . . . . . . . . . . . . . . . . . . . . . . . . . . . . . .90
                    Sidebar: Don't Blow A Fuse! . . . . . . . . . . . . . . . . . . . . . . . . . . . . . . . . . .90
                Vitamins and Minerals . . . . . . . . . . . . . . . . . . . . . . . . . . . . . . . . . . . . . . . . .91
                    *Immnunonutrition: Using Supplements Sensibly, by Dr. Alice Villalobos* . . . . . . . . *92*
                Supplements . . . . . . . . . . . . . . . . . . . . . . . . . . . . . . . . . . . . . . . . . . . . . . . .94
                Alternative Therapies . . . . . . . . . . . . . . . . . . . . . . . . . . . . . . . . . . . . . . . . . .97

        Bullet's Supplements . . . . . . . . . . . . . . . . . . . . . . . . . . . . . . . . . . . . . . . . .97

        Assessing Success . . . . . . . . . . . . . . . . . . . . . . . . . . . . . . . . . . . . . . . . . .99

CHAPTER 9    **Whole Health** . . . . . . . . . . . . . . . . . . . . . . . . . . . . . . . . . . . . . . . . . . . . .**101**

        Weak Spots with Cancer . . . . . . . . . . . . . . . . . . . . . . . . . . . . . . . . . . . .102

        Vaccines and Cancer . . . . . . . . . . . . . . . . . . . . . . . . . . . . . . . . . . . . . .106

        Other Preventives . . . . . . . . . . . . . . . . . . . . . . . . . . . . . . . . . . . . . . . . .106

           *Vaccines and Canine Cancer Patients, by Dr. W. Jean Dodds* . . . . . . . . . . . . . .*107*

        Be Prepared . . . . . . . . . . . . . . . . . . . . . . . . . . . . . . . . . . . . . . . . . . . .109

CHAPTER 10   **From Warriors to Angels** . . . . . . . . . . . . . . . . . . . . . . . . . . . . . . . . . . . . .**111**

        When Pawspice Begins . . . . . . . . . . . . . . . . . . . . . . . . . . . . . . . . . . . .112

        When Pawspice Ends . . . . . . . . . . . . . . . . . . . . . . . . . . . . . . . . . . . . .113

        After The Loss . . . . . . . . . . . . . . . . . . . . . . . . . . . . . . . . . . . . . . . . . .115

        Measuring Grief . . . . . . . . . . . . . . . . . . . . . . . . . . . . . . . . . . . . . . . . .116

   **Bullet's Story, Part Two: Epilogue** . . . . . . . . . . . . . . . . . . . . . . . . . . . . . . .**121**

        So Easy to Love, So Hard to Lose: Bullet's Eulogy . . . . . . . . . . . . . . . . . . . 129

   References . . . . . . . . . . . . . . . . . . . . . . . . . . . . . . . . . . . . . . . . . . . . . . 131

   Resources . . . . . . . . . . . . . . . . . . . . . . . . . . . . . . . . . . . . . . . . . . . . . . . 133

   Vaccination Waiver Request . . . . . . . . . . . . . . . . . . . . . . . . . . . . . . . . . . . 136

   "Early Warning Signs of Cancer and Illness" Poster . . . . . . . . . . . . . . . . . . . . . . 137

   **The Magic Bullet Fund** . . . . . . . . . . . . . . . . . . . . . . . . . . . . . . . . . . . . . . .**139**

# WITH GRATITUDE

I was very lucky to have the support of many special people in and around the creation of this book, beginning with Bullet's top-notch medical team. The excellent care that Bullet received before, during and after cancer was the foundation for his long survival and, hence, for this book.

Bullet's primary-care team, Dr. Bruce Hoskins and the entire Croton Animal Hospital staff, kept him healthy and strong throughout and were ever tolerant of Bullet's antics (and my own). For expert emergency care, I thank Dr. Chris Angiello, Dr. Joe Impellizeri and the wonderful staff at the Katonah-Bedford Veterinary Center, Bedford Hills, NY as well as the Foster Small Animal Hospital at Tufts.

The expertise of Bullet's cancer team is self-evident in light of his long survival, particularly Dr. Paolo Porzio, who also envisioned this book long before I was ready to write it. Veterinary oncologist Dr. David Ruslander provided invaluable guidance during Bullet's treatment in all cancer-related matters, and other health issues as well. He also contributed to your dog's well-being by reviewing the content of this book for medical accuracy.

Holistic veterinarians Dr. Bea Ehrsam, Dr. Tina Aiken and Dr. Marty Goldstein expanded on our home care plan to include a holistic dimension. All components of Bullet's home care program evolved from their initial recommendations the week of his diagnosis.

Important contributions to this book were made by veterinary oncologists Dr. Phil Bergman, Dr. Kevin Hahn and Dr. Rodney Page. Each composed a page with an informative and heartfelt message for the readers of this book. This book would be conspicuously lacking were it not for the contributions of veterinarians Dr. W. Jean Dodds, who shares her extensive knowledge of vaccines; and Dr. Alice Villalobos, who shares some vital information about supplementation.

I owe my eternal gratitude to Karen Summers for her unending patience, her sense of humor and her extensive assistance in the many tasks required to produce this second edition of Help Your Dog Fight Cancer. Karen is a volunteer for the Magic Bullet Fund as well, with her Siberian, Tensing, in treatment for lymphoma. During the past 8 months, Karen's dedication to the fund has been invaluable and is appreciated by myself and everyone affiliated with the fund.

I must express my heartfelt gratitude to Bullet's many wonderful "Aunts and Uncles," who provided emotional support to me and hands-on care for Bullet over the years: Tracy Basile, Kevin Griffin, Andrea Rabe, Catriona and Dave Lappell and Connie Schwarting, Rick and Abby Kaplan (Bullet's actual Uncle and Aunt), Lynn and Ron Schwager (Bullet's Godparents), Janet Kaplan (grandmother) and Margot and Dick Basile (his adopted grandparents). Thank you all for being there for me and Bullet, through thick and thin!

Last, but not least, I thank you! I cringe with every new book order—another dog has cancer. Nonetheless, I am gratified that another dog will benefit from Bullet's ordeal and that another person will keep Bullet's memory alive. This book is a labor of love, for Bullet and for your dog as well.

# INTRODUCTION

*by Bruce N. Hoskins, DVM*

As a veterinarian in companion animal practice for more than fifteen years, I have encountered many challenging cases and experienced, alongside my clients, many difficult losses. To me, however, the most difficult task I have to perform is that of informing a client their beloved pet has a disease that may prematurely end that pet's life.

Anyone fortunate enough to have experienced the unconditional love of a pet understands the mutual devotion that this relationship can foster and the profound sadness and distress that comes with news of a terminal illness. When the diagnosis is cancer, I see an added element of stress, stemming from the fear and frustration of dealing with the unknown.

Most of us have been touched in some way by human cancer. We know of some people who have succumbed to the disease or to treatment and others who are surviving. In contrast, most of my clients whose pets have cancer do *not* have a personal resource for information and support. Most do not have a friend who has seen their pet through cancer treatment. Through this book, Laurie has become that friend to many people.

I treated Bullet for many conditions over the past 12 years, ranging from the basic annual exam to Lyme Disease, bite wounds from altercations with other dogs and bone chips in his shoulder

joint. He was a good patient, aside from the growls and complaints typical of the breed. Laurie was very much the devoted "mother," seeing Bullet through those spectacles of adoration that we all wear when we look at our pets. Still, she has always responded to treatment recommendations

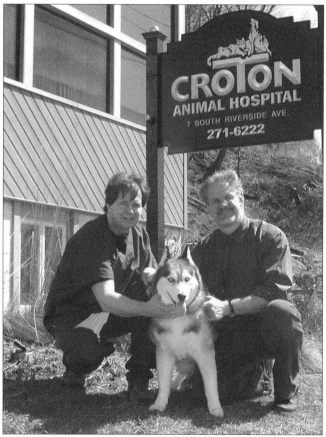

From left: Vet Tech Ed Mowan, Bullet, Dr. Bruce Hoskins

with thoughtful consideration and objectivity. These are important elements for the caretaker of a canine cancer patient to develop in order to become an effective advocate.

Some clients are reluctant to ask questions and become passive observers of their pet's cancer treatment. The author of this book is decidedly not in that client group. Laurie asks all of the questions that I expect a client might ask, and then goes on to ask more.

Laurie has been a true advocate for Bullet in every sense of the word. She went to great lengths to educate herself about Bullet's diagnosis, treatment options, home-care options and potential complications. She challenged each and every member of Bullet's cancer team to research the hard questions and to "think outside the box" in order to find solutions for Bullet.

I have been changed by my experience with Bullet and Laurie, especially during the four-plus years since Bullet's cancer diagnosis. He was my first patient to beat the odds and become a canine lymphoma survivor. Laurie never once lost faith in Bullet's ability to overcome cancer and, on more than one occasion, to survive severe treatment side effects and secondary complications. Through my relationship with Bullet and Laurie, I acquired a new respect for the power of a positive outlook and a team approach to the cancer fight, centered on the active involvement of the caretaker.

Veterinarians have written texts about canine cancer to be read by veterinarians. A few have written books for caretakers. Notably missing was a book written by a caretaker, for caretakers. In *Help Your Dog Fight Cancer*, Laurie offers a great deal of information and support, but even more valuable is that she strives to empower caretakers to become their dog's advocate and an active member of the cancer team.

In July of 2000, I had the task of delivering a diagnosis of multicentric lymphoma in Bullet. It was a sad day, but it was the beginning of what was to become a poignant success story of canine cancer survival.

In November 2004, Bullet died, never having come out of remission from lymphoma. Bullet's triumph against cancer has produced a legacy through which he will help many caretakers to help their dogs fight cancer. I am happy to have been a part of Bullet's cancer team and to have been able to work with him and his devoted human companion, Laurie Kaplan.

*Bruce N. Hoskins, DVM, is the owner of and a practitioner at the three-veterinarian small animal practice, Croton Animal Hospital, in Croton-on-Hudson, NY.*

# Author's Foreword

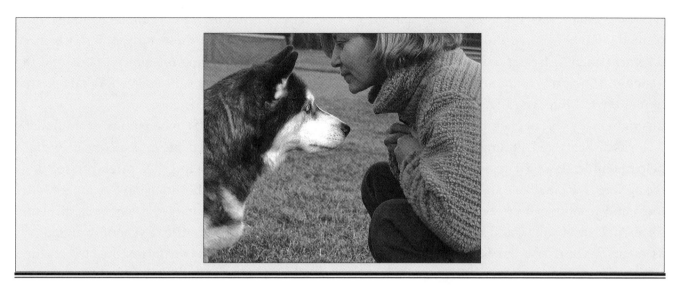

Experts predict that approximately half of our dogs will have cancer in their lifetimes and yet, as caretakers, most of us know little or nothing about caring for a dog with cancer. Not long ago, admittedly, there wasn't much to know. Today, however, treatment for canine cancer is nearly on a par with treatment for human cancer and there is a great deal to know.

If your dog has cancer, you're undoubtedly asking, *"What can I do?"* First, you'll see that a medical plan is decided upon and put into action. This book will help you to decide on a plan and to decide how active a role you will play in your dog's fight against cancer. You'll read about the treatment options for canine cancer and the types of decisions that you can be involved in making right from the start. Whatever degree of involvement you choose, *Help Your Dog Fight Cancer* will help you on your way.

Once a medical plan has been decided upon, you'll ask, *"What else can I do?"* Lots! Regardless of what type of medical treatment you choose (chemotherapy, radiation, surgery, an alternative therapy or no treatment at all), there is a great deal more that you can do. You'll learn how to manage symptoms and side effects, strengthen your dog's organs and bolster his system. You'll learn how to help your dog better fight the disease and better tolerate the treatment and perhaps you'll improve his odds for survival.

When Bullet was diagnosed with cancer, I wanted to know what could, might and typically does happen in such cases. I wanted to know what I should, shouldn't, could and might do to help him survive. Moreover, I wanted to know all of this right away and in plain English.

I was disheartened, finding no book that would help me understand the typical course of events, the options, the possible pitfalls, how to deal with them and what to expect—best case and worst. I set about learning all I could as quickly as I could, as many devoted and terrified cancer-dog caretakers have done in recent years. My experience as an animal writer and editor of medical literature hadn't educated me about canine cancer in any way that would be helpful to me as the caretaker of a cancer dog, but did enable me to wade through medical literature reasonably undaunted by medical lingo and to write this book.

During the first year of Bullet's cancer treatment, I consulted general practice veterinarians, veterinary oncologists, holistic vets, oncologists in human medicine and other caretakers of dogs with cancer. I read books both medical and lay to research medications, supplements, nutraceuticals, diets and clinical trials. I experimented extensively to find the regimen that would work best for both Bullet and me.

The more information I gathered and the more I understood about Bullet's condition, the more capable I felt of caring for him properly and the more my anxiety level diminished. What research didn't teach me, experience did.

Paolo Porzio, DVM, who administered Bullet's chemotherapy, urged me repeatedly to write a book that would help other caretakers of dogs with cancer allay those feelings of anxiety that come from not knowing—the very book that I had not been able to find. After a year of shrugging off Dr. Porzio's urgings, I finally resigned my position as editor-in-chief of *Catnip* magazine, a publication of Tufts University School of Veterinary Medicine, and set about writing this book.

For Bullet's sake, I researched and fact-checked while choosing options for his care. For your dog's sake, I did more research and fact checking while composing this book. Wherever possible, I provide the source of my data. Much of it, however, has been accumulated from undocumented sources or is based on my own experience.

The three key members of Bullet's team—his general practice veterinarian, the doctor who provided chemotherapy and the veterinary oncologist who served as our consultant—have all been kind enough to fact-check the manuscript of *Help Your Dog Fight Cancer* for medical accuracy and to ensure that, according to what is now known about canine cancer, no recommendations are made that might harm a cancer dog.

Several top-notch veterinarians and veterinary oncologists have each generously composed a page to *Help Your Dog Fight Cancer* in their area of expertise or special interest. No one of these experts agrees with every facet of Bullet's home-care program or every recommendation presented in this book.

As you develop a home-care regimen for your dog, discuss your plans with your veterinarian. Include any facets of Bullet's home-care program that you wish to use. Some methods that have worked well for Bullet could be contraindicated for your dog's breed or condition, the type of cancer that he has, his individual sensitivities or the medical treatment he's receiving.

I've helped many caretakers begin the bittersweet journey involved in living with and caring for a cancer dog. All are initially overwhelmed, as I was, by the endless list of decisions to be made. *Help Your Dog Fight Cancer* doesn't contain an encyclopedic listing of treatments, supplements, dosages and diets. Rather, it presents the "short list" for each and then shares the shorter list that defines the choices I've made over the years in building a home-care program for my cancer dog.

There are a thousand different ways to care for a dog with cancer and each caretaker has to choose his or her options. I offer no evidence that the care package I've designed for Bullet is responsible for his survival. Without chemotherapy, Bullet would certainly have had no chance of survival longer than the typical four to six week period predicted for dogs with untreated lymphoma. It may be that Bullet's survival so far beyond his prognosis was simply his hardy constitution and his extremely stubborn personality.

My hope is that every reader will come away from *Help Your Dog Fight Cancer* with a plan and with confidence, prepared to begin the journey. Be creative, flexible, adventurous and careful in caring for your cancer dog. And keep the faith!

In caring for my cancer dog and in composing this book, I've taken great pains to discover those treatments and therapies that I believe to have the greatest potential for success from a variety of sources within traditional and holistic medicine.

Cancer is a fierce enemy, and to "fight the good fight," we need all the ammunition we can get. *Help Your Dog Fight Cancer* will provide you with a solid foundation for your battle against canine cancer. Armed with information and love, you will discover the best possible way to care for your own cancer dog.

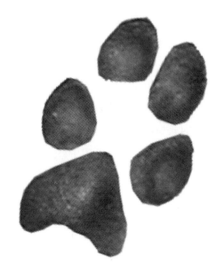

## PAWPRINTS

The pawprints in this book are not generic. When I completed the first edition of this book, I attempted to hold Bullet's arm, press his foot onto a (non-toxic) ink pad, and press his paw on the title page. He was clearly not going to agree to this.

I shot a digital photo of the bottom of Bullet's foot and used a photo editor to remove everything except the pads. These are the next best thing to Bullet's actual pawprint. If your dog has cancer, I hope he will follow in Bullet's big pawprints.

# BULLET'S STORY, PART ONE

*Prologue*

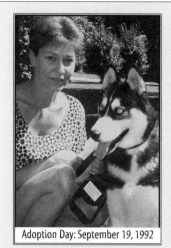

Adoption Day: September 19, 1992

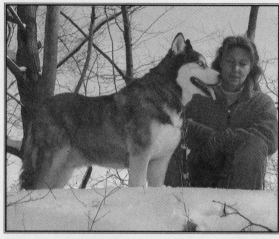

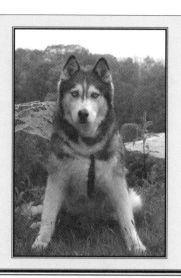

I must take this opportunity to tell Bullet's story and to claim for him the "15 minutes of fame" that is most certainly his due. If your dog has been diagnosed with cancer and you are feeling overwhelmed, please skip this Prologue and go directly to Chapter 1.

I'd lived with cats for many years—15 cats in all, but never more than three at a time for fear of earning the title "the cat lady." I was toying with the idea of sharing my home with a dog in addition to my three resident felines, KC, Bumi and TipToe. On September 19, 1992, I wandered into the local animal shelter from which I had adopted TipToe a year earlier, intending only to hand out biscuits to the pups and explore my feelings about bringing a new member, of the canine species, into the family.

My friend Kevin and I perused the canine residents, handed out biscuits to many and took a few for walks in the shelter parking lot. Then, Kevin pointed out a dog in one of the large kennels. The ID tag hanging on the cage indicated that this was Max, an 18-month-old neutered male Siberian Husky. Max was sitting quietly amidst the chaos generated by several other medium-to-large dogs who cohabited the cage, all barking wildly and vying for position to receive biscuits.

Max had the most beautiful ears and eyes I'd ever seen. He was strikingly black and white with a handsome star-shaped design on his chest. I looked at Max and he looked at me. It was a bit unnerving, being studied with such intensity by two icy blue eyes in a canine head. Love at first sight? Maybe so—in any case, I knew then and there that this dog with super-canine eye contact was going to be mine.

According to the shelter manager, the dog had just been relinquished by his owner the previous day. The owner complained that Max was an escape artist and a "runner." He had had to retrieve Max from dog control one time too many.

I've since learned, by reading up on the breed and by chasing Bullet down many, many times, that it's redundant to say a dog is a Siberian Husky *and* a runner. In fact, I had an opportunity to witness the Siberian penchant for escape early on. I had Max taken from his kennel and walked him around the parking lot. I then left Kevin holding the leash and I went into the office to pay the suggested $40 donation. When I came out a few minutes later, I found Kevin still holding the leash...only now the leash was dangling to the ground with no dog attached to it. "Oh," Kevin said when he noticed my expression. "You're *taking* that dog?"

A shelter worker, my friend Kevin and I all set out to chase Max down. He seemed to be having great fun watching the three of us over his shoulder and eluding our attempts at capture. Finally, exasperated, I stopped running, clapped my hands and yelled *"MAAAAX!"* To everyone's amazement, Max ran right to me from behind a nearby house and rolled over on his back at my feet—an event that would never ever happen again.

Soon thereafter, "Max" became "Bullet" (as in faster than a speeding...) because of his great love of running. His friends call him "Bully" because of his great love of growling.

During our first six months together, Bullet was ousted from three boarding kennels and two dog trainers proclaimed him untrainable. One went so far as to recommend that I return him to the shelter...alas, it was too late. I suspect it was too late from the moment that I put him into my car at the shelter.

Bullet destroyed everything that was not nailed down, and a few things that were. He loved nothing more than to chew on (never bite) a human hand or arm. Periodically, I went in another room and closed the door to give myself a "time out" from Bullet. I was exhausted from yelling "NO!" over and over. I came across the movie, Turner and Hooch and howled with laughter—I related completely to Turner's (played by Tom Hanks) frustration and exasperation.

As a strong healthy youth, Bullet was a big-time puller "on leash." If only I had a nickel for every time a passer-by said *"Who's walking who?"* I didn't weigh much more than Bullet and he was quite capable of pulling me right off my feet—especially if a squirrel, rabbit or cat happened by to provide incentive.

When Bullet encountered unfamiliar dogs, he always became extremely agitated and I was never entirely sure whether he intended to play or fight. I would drag him off-trail, grab onto a tree and hang on until the dog passed by. But he loved all people and was always happy to allow anyone and everyone to pet him and admire him.

True to the breed, Bullet ran away whenever possible. He could chew through a nylon or leather leash so quickly and surreptitiously that he would be on the run with a healthy head start by the time I realized that he wasn't at the end of the leash. He even managed to get away from one of the dog trainers who worked with him. Come to think of it, that was the same trainer who had suggested that I return Bullet to the shelter!

I knew there was nothing wrong with this dog that a lot of tender love (and a lot of *tough* love) couldn't fix. I read dog-training books and books about the Husky personality. What I needed was a how-to book for training a Siberian Husky.

After a few months, a few books and a few new wrinkles on my brow, Bullet became a bit more manageable. After a few years of training (what one friend calls "Laurie's Boot Camp"), Bullet and I found a place of mutual respect with me as the Alpha (albeit by a slim margin). Bullet was a ridiculously high maintenance dog. In time, he became a very opinionated but manageable dog. The older he got, the better he got and later, in his geriatric years, he was darn near perfect.

Bullet mastered basic obedience commands such as Sit, Down, Stay, Paw, Other Paw, Jump, Speak and Kiss (this last was always our favorite), but he never ever learned to "Come" off lead. I'm quite sure it's an auditory problem—Bullet's hearing is just fine with a leash attached, but he reliably goes stone-cold deaf the moment the leash is clicked off from the collar. From my readings and from talking to other frustrated and bemused Siberian caretakers, I gather this hearing problem is genetic and breed-related.

At first, Bullet slept in a finished basement at night. I had planned to introduce him to the cats gradually before allowing him free run of the house. I would go downstairs each morning to find the floor littered with remnants of books, notepads, computer disks, pencils and anything else within his reach. My friend Joe Mullins, who had lived with Malamutes, convinced me that because Bullet was a Northern-breed dog, he should sleep outdoors. In light of the wreckage, this sounded to me like a great idea.

So Bullet moved to the great outdoors, with his collar hooked onto an overhead run between two trees 50 feet apart. He had a doghouse full of hay but always chose to sleep under the stars, except in the most inclement weather. In lightening and thunderstorms, he slept indoors because outdoor dogs can be struck by lightening.

During the winter, a dog's tongue can tear on frozen-over water. I had an electrical outlet installed next to the doghouse and purchased a heated water bowl. To make further use of the outlet, I plugged in a baby monitor and placed it in the doghouse. Its counterpart hung beside my bed. More often than I care to remember, I was awakened in the wee hours by frantic barking coming through my end of the baby monitor. De-skunking baths in the front yard at 2 a.m. became commonplace, followed by a car ride in search of a dumpster while holding a multi-wrapped skunk carcass out of the window as far as possible from my nose.

In 1995, I installed a 5-foot high chain-link fence in the woods behind my house. The resulting dog pen measured 50 feet by 50 feet—larger than the footprint of my house. Furnished with a doghouse, lounge chair and flat-roofed eating station, this pen gave Bullet freedom from the overhead run, put a stop to the skunk carnage and became "Bully's World."

Bullet taught me how to train an "untrainable" dog. He taught me to understand dog-speak and to communicate with him in a way that he could understand. But he taught me much more than this. For example, Bullet inspired me to learn to knit so that I could make sweaters, vests and scarves from his fur.

Dog fur becomes quite fuzzy when knitted, looking very much like mohair, and the final product is so warm that I was unable to wear my Bully-sweaters indoors. I turned sweaters into vests by removing the sleeves and, so as not to waste any precious fur, I turned the detached sleeves into slipper-socks.

Bullet taught me to mush. On winter weekends, we went on dog sledding trips in Lake Placid, NY. There, he added a few new commands to his repertoire: Hike (start running), Gee (turn right), Haw (turn left), Straight On and Whoa. On these weekend trips, usually with my friend Kevin, I rented a cabin and a sled and three Huskies from the owner of a professional Siberian dog sledding team. What a rush! Seeing Bullet take to sledding like a duck to water gave me new respect for who he was and for the natural order of things.

Bullet acquired a new nickname when friend Tracy Basile visited an American Indian Reservation. On her return, she was inspired to assign new names to our dogs. Her dogs, Kai (lion-hearted deer-dog, friend of the coyotes) and Toshi (frog-dancer, water-prancer) were Bullet's best furry friends for many years. During a solemn naming ceremony, we appropriately dubbed my very ornery little boy "Bullet Growly Bear."

Tracy and I contracted a trainer to work with Bullet, Kai and Toshi once a week, teaching them (and us) agility as well as reinforcing and refining their basic obedience. Inez added Jump, Tunnel and Hoop to Bullet's vocabulary.

When Bullet was 7, he had arthroscopic surgery on both shoulders to remove a bone chip and debris from the joints. This marked the end of Bullet's sledding days and squashed any fantasies I may have had of running in the Iditarod.

By then, two of my cats had died at ripe old ages. The third, TipToe, packed her bags and moved next door to stay with a friend and neighbor. I wanted Bullet to recuperate indoors, without re-injuring his shoulders chasing TipToe. TipToe and Margaret fell in love and shared a home for

eight years, until Margaret went to the Rainbow Bridge at 91 years of age. When TipToe moved next door, Bullet became a house dog, and he made this transition without complaint.

Bullet's recovery from his shoulder surgery was difficult. My unruly, rebellious and fiercely independent dog had become dependent.

Bullet did regain his strength and his air of independence, but lost a bit of his craziness. He was (finally) a mature dog. He liked to lie under the table during weekly bridge games, waiting for someone to offer him a pizza crust during dinner. He loved to greet visitors at the door and was always very happy to wrestle with anyone willing to endure his mock-vicious growls and attacks.

## THE DIAGNOSIS

In May 2000, I felt enlarged nodes in Bullet's neck, just where a doctor will feel your neck if you complain of a sore throat. Initially, our veterinarian suspected allergies and prescribed antihistamines. But the enlarged nodes remained in spite of the medications.

Bullet's lifelong primary care veterinarian, Bruce Hoskins, DVM, at Croton Animal Hospital in Croton-on-Hudson, NY, attempted a needle biopsy of a lymph node in order to rule out lymphoma. The fluid that was extracted did not contain lymph fluid and so a surgical biopsy was performed the following day.

Dr. Hoskins took the biopsy sample from the popliteal lymph node behind Bullet's left knee. The node had all but disintegrated during the procedure, he said, and had to be excised entirely. Dr. Hoskins said that it might be lymphoma, but if so, he thought it was a very early stage cancer.

The next evening, on July 17, 2000, Dr. Hoskins called to say, "The laboratory report on Bullet's biopsy was positive for lymphoma." I knew that this could not be true. *There must be a mistake.* Aside from the swollen glands I'd found in his neck, Bullet was a strong, healthy 9-year-old Siberian Husky. Physically and behaviorally, he emitted an air of strength, health and heartiness and seemed impervious to illness and injury. Surely, the laboratory got their blood samples mixed up or had misinterpreted the results. "No," I was assured, "there is no mistake."

I was dumfounded. I was shocked. I had a lump in my throat and a knot in my stomach. I stayed up all night, intermittently hugging him, crying, researching canine lymphoma online and contacting anyone and everyone I knew in the field of veterinary medicine or cancer research for advice. I was, at that time, editor-in-chief of a med-

ical newsmagazine called *Catnip*, a publication from Tufts University School of Veterinary Medicine. The show of support from the top-notch Tufts veterinarians when they learned of Bullet's illness touched, impressed and strengthened me.

Dr. Hoskins provided the names and telephone numbers of local veterinary oncologists and a local veterinarian who was not board certified in oncology but provided cancer treatment to dogs and cats. This was Dr. Paolo Porzio. In July 2000, luckily for us, he was at the Tuckahoe Animal Hospital in Tuckahoe, NY, just half an hour away.

Dr. Porzio agreed to start Bullet on chemotherapy the very next day. At first, I chose him to begin Bullet's treatment based on location and availability despite the fact that he was not board certified in oncology. The most important thing, in my mind, was to get Bullet into treatment as quickly as possible.

During our very first visit, however, I knew that Dr. Porzio was a great choice. He was very attentive to Bullet during our conversation and spoke to him in a sweet, gentle and affectionate way. His "bedside manner" was perfect. He spoke clearly, explained everything to me in an unrushed manner and took his time answering all of my many questions thoroughly. Also, his veterinary clinic was on the ground floor and the storefront was a huge plate-glass window. Before entering, I could see if there were any dogs in the waiting room—a big plus, since Bullet didn't always take kindly to new dogs. It was a relief to know that there would never be a ruckus in the waiting room or a struggle to keep Bullet from lunging at another dog.

Dr. Porzio had completed a residency in internal medicine in Saskatchewan. There was no staff oncologist at the school at the time, so the class had to learn to provide cancer treatment for the local dogs. The location appealed to me because not all doctors are enamored of the exuberance and obstinance of the Siberian Husky. In Saskatchewan, Dr. Porzio would have become familiar with the many idiosyncrasies and antics of the breed.

Dr. Porzio treated cancer dogs using a single-agent (one drug) chemotherapy protocol using an agent called doxorubicin. I read about this drug and consulted several veterinary oncologists, most notably Dr. Dave Ruslander. At that time Dr. Ruslander was at Tufts Veterinary School and he recommended a treatment plan called VELCAP-L for Bullet. This was a more complex protocol, but showed a higher success rate than the single-agent doxorubicin protocol. Dr. Porzio readily agreed to use the VELCAP-L treatment plan for Bullet with Dr. Ruslander's guidance. Dr. Ruslander con-

tributed immeasurably to Bullet's well-being and survival over the years.

Once I had a medical treatment plan in place, I wanted to know, *"What else can I do?"* I made an appointment with a local holistic vet, who spoke to me of many cancer dogs who had survived and attributed their survival to the treatment that he had provided. He gave me my first lesson in holistic cancer support. I had been so eager and determined to see this guru of holistic pet care that I didn't even bother to find out the cost of the consultation. After the appointment was over, I was handed a bill for over $750.00, and was told that all of the veterinarians at the clinic provide the same treatment and information, but at a fraction of the cost.

At this point I was off and running and ready to settle in for what I hoped would be a long haul. The initial panic and fear subsided and I prepared to do my part in perpetually fine tuning Bullet's treatment and home care and spend the remainder of my free time just loving his company, handling glitches that popped up and treasuring every single moment of borrowed time with my beautiful boy.

Bullet's Story continues on page 121.

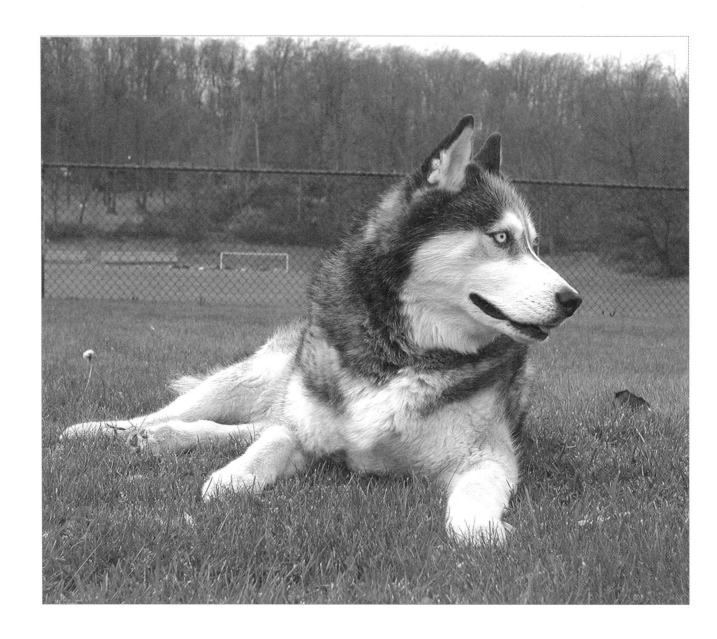

# PREPARE FOR BATTLE

*You may wage war against the beast that threatens*
*To take the life of your companion.*
*Choose your weapons and*
*Recruit fearless warriors*
*into your army.*
*But even in the midst of battle,*
*Take time to peel away the warrior,*
*To reveal a soft heart, to give a gentle touch,*
*To treasure every precious moment of borrowed time.*

"*our dog has cancer.*" Suddenly, your pal, your playful companion, hiking buddy, confidante and protector (or protectee) has become a cancer patient. You no longer look at him with eyes full of happiness and love. Your eyes, your tone of voice, your posture and your energy all speak of sadness, pity, fear and anger.

Dogs are sensitive to the type of energy (vibes) that their humans project. Don't let your long face be a "downer" for your dog when he's ill, and especially not when he's feeling well and happy. When a caretaker is upset, a dog wonders what he's done wrong. My message is not to *put on* a happy face, but to actually *have* a happy face and

a happy heart. Hold him close and let his fur absorb your tears on occasion. But, for the main, stay upbeat and positive and be grateful and full of joy for the time that he has been with you and because he's with you now. Thoroughly relish every day that you have together and keep reminding yourself that your best friend is now on borrowed time. Each day is a precious gift.

*"How can I pretend to be happy when I'm so sad?"* Don't pretend! Tend to your dog, do whatever you can to make him comfortable and focus your attention on working to pull him through. Use your imagination—even the smallest contributions that you make to improve his comfort level are very important.

When you've done everything you can and there's nothing more to do, simply sit by his side, pet him, sing him a song! Bullet proved to me that dogs like being sung to even if the singer can't carry a tune. If singing is out of the question, then talk to your dog or read him a poem! The sound of your voice will soothe him. Remember to say his name often.

Without chemotherapy, dogs with lymphoma generally perish within a month. The accuracy of this prognosis varies, depending on how long the disease was present before diagnosis. Dr. Ruslander, DVM, diplomate ACVIM (Oncology), diplomate ACVR (Radiation Oncology), at the Veterinary Specialty Hospital of the Carolinas in Cary, NC, was Bullet's oncology consultant. Dr. Ruslander said that, with chemotherapy, 50 percent of dogs with lymphoma survive one year and 25 percent survive two years or more.

I was afraid to hope that Bullet might be lucky enough to fall into this minority. I liked the sound of a one-year remission, though, because Bullet was just past his ninth birthday when diagnosed. A one-year reprieve would afford him a normal life span for a Siberian Husky.

In July of 2000, Bullet had his first visit with Paolo Porzio, DVM, diplomate ACVIM (internal medicine), who now practices in Mississauga, Ontario, Canada. The doctor said that he thought Bullet would be very happy when the weather turned cold. I asked (dubiously) if he really thought Bullet would still be here by the next snowfall. He was still here, not only for the entire next winter, but for the next four winters! Many dogs survive various types of cancer for long periods of time. Some enjoy a normal life span and live on, to die years later from a completely unrelated cause.

## NOT TODAY

Be strong, for your dog's sake and your own. We each have a different method of fortifying ourselves emotionally. When you feel overwhelmed or emotionally exhausted, gather strength from talking to sympathetic family and friends about your journey. Make use of your support system. Take a break from researching. Sit by your dog and do nothing but stroke him for a while. Say: *Not today, and not without a fight!*

When it comes to death and dying, dogs are blessed with ignorance. They don't know that they may die soon or that they have a disease called cancer. Dogs don't regret or complain about what happened yesterday, nor do they anticipate or fear what might happen tomorrow. We humans are not so lucky. We know, we fear, we anticipate and we project. While caring for your cancer dog, shed your natural inclination to dwell on these emotions—to fret over yesterday's decisions or worry about what tomorrow will bring.

Be in the moment—emulate your dog! It's is an ongoing process to maintain this attitude. Every time Bullet went through a bad spell, I wondered if, and hoped that, he was going to recover "this time." I reminded myself, over and over, to remain calm, treat the symptoms and hope for the best. The journey is an emotionally exhausting roller coaster ride. So hang on tight and keep saying "Not Today and Not Without a Fight!"

# KEEP A LOG

If you're a journal writer, sharpen your pencil! If not, do your best to keep a simple list of notable events. The information in your log may very well save your dog from having to endure side effects unnecessarily. A few months into treatment, you may find yourself trying to remember, *"Which agent was it that caused that terrible reaction?"* or *"How long was it before my dog was feeling better the last time this happened?"* or *"What were his symptoms and which remedy was it that finally alleviated those symptoms?"*

ITEMS TO INCLUDE IN YOUR LOG

‣ Medications and supplements given
‣ Any change in diet
‣ Any change in eating, urination and defecation habits or mood
‣ Names and dates of treatments (including a printout of the protocol being used)
‣ Side effects and reactions
‣ All attempts to counteract side effects
‣ What worked and what didn't
‣ How long it took for the remedy to resolve the problem
‣ Which team member (or other source) suggested the remedy
‣ Secondary illnesses

The simple notations in your log could help you get a repeat episode under control quickly. Veterinarians you consult may ask you for information such as when you started giving your dog a particular medication or supplement, at what dose and how he responded. If your log contains the answers, it will help the doctor make the most effective recommendations without delay.

Look into a valuable service provided by Pet Summary. Record your dog's medical history online, where it can be accessed any time, by any veterinarian. [www.PetSummary.com]

# Don't Be Afraid To Ask

How much medical information do you want? Some people just find it all too complicated and would rather put the problem in the doctor's hands and leave it at that. As a result, many medical doctors and veterinarians comply—they don't volunteer extensive medical information because they don't expect their patients/clients to be interested or to participate in the decision-making process.

If "medicalese" is Greek to you and you want to keep it that way, ask your veterinarian to consult a specialist—a board certified veterinary oncologist. Members of this small and elite group of experts are aware of the most up to date data about canine cancer care. With the assistance of your veterinarian and a specialist, you will design a solid treatment plan for your dog.

If you *do* want to know and you *do* want to play a role in deciding on a treatment plan, make very sure that your veterinarian is aware of this. Don't passively nod "okay" when he outlines a plan. Rather, ask him to outline all of the options and to explain why he chose the treatment plan that he did. Tell your veterinarian that, with his guidance, you will make all final decisions about your dog's care. Talk to other veterinarians, consult specialists and anyone you can think of who can contribute to your knowledge bank about

## No Contract

A decision to begin cancer treatment for your dog does not in any way obligate you to continue treatment ad infinitum. When making this decision, keep in mind that there is no contract—you can stop treatment at any time.

It's always difficult to call it quits, but it's even more difficult to keep an unhappy animal alive when there's no real hope for a turnaround. A decline in the dog's quality of life is always a good and compelling reason to stop treatment.

People often discontinue cancer treatment because their dog isn't responding to treatment or becomes dangerously ill from it. Others stop due to financial constraints.

There's nothing wrong with giving your dog an extra 3, 5 or 7 months of life (and also giving yourself those additional months to spend with him) and then choosing a stopping point when the financial outlay has reached a certain limit.

Take the pressure off! If you're unable to make a long-term decision, keep your options open by providing treatment until you're able to decide. If you withhold treatment and later decide to treat, the time lost may diminish the chances of success.

canine cancer. As your dog's first advocate, make the best decision you can and don't look back.

Also remember to ask your veterinarians for copies of all blood test, laboratory and surgical reports. Keep these in a file for easy reference.

Join an online support group! The members generally do not have veterinary degrees but they know a great deal and are willing to share their knowledge and support.

Tensing, a Siberian with lymphoma, was in chemotherapy. After about ten treatments, his veterinarian told his caretaker that Tensing was in remission and, therefore, did not need to continue treatment. When a chemotherapy protocol is not completed, remission may end. Tensing did come out of remission and his caretaker called me for assistance. Tensing became a Magic Bullet Fund dog and treatment was started anew.

Tensing was kept overnight after every chemo treatment. He was having 18-hour infusions of chemotherapy, left in a clinic kennel, unattended throughout the night. A support group would have told Tensing's caretaker that treatments take between 20 minutes and 2 hours, and that it's very risky to abandon a protocol midstream.

I was dreading the day Bullet would come out of remission. *"How will I know? When might it be? What will happen next?"* That feeling of being unprepared, of not knowing what to expect, was creating anxiety. The solution was to get some hard cold facts, so, I asked.

Dr. Porzio said Bullet's lymph nodes would suddenly become enlarged. *"Might I miss it?"* "Like golf balls!" he said. He showed me where these golf balls would appear. I began to check for lymph node enlargement every day—I suggest you do the same. You can disguise the check as a petting/massaging session! Scratch the top of his head, tweak the ears, run your fingers down his back along the spine... and add a check of the loca-

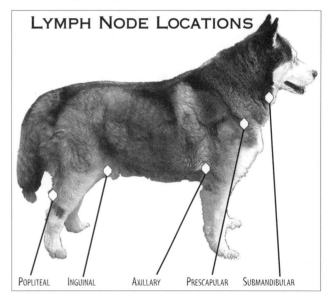

Lymph node enlargement is often the first sign of cancer and the first sign of a relapsed remission. Check your dog's lymph nodes regularly. (Of course, there's a matching set on left side of the dog.)

tions where the nodes reside. I stopped daily checks a year after Bullet's chemotherapy ended, but I continued to check them once a week.

Dr. Porzio and I discussed various rescue therapies used for dogs relapsing from a remission. We agreed that, if and when Bullet came out of remission, we would call on our board certified veterinary oncologist consultant, for guidance.

Be very clear about what the signs will be if and when your dog comes out of remission. Ask your oncologist to show you exactly where you will see or feel a change and what it will look like. The first sign of a failed remission is often enlarged lymph nodes (see "Lymph Node Locator, on page 13). Feel the nodes regularly and make a note of their sizes. Inform your doctor immediately if the nodes suddenly feel larger.

Apart from enlarged lymph nodes, Bullet was asymptomatic at the time of his diagnosis. This is often the case, especially with lymphoma. During the year and a half that followed, Bullet became ill many times. I knew that it was the treatment, not the cancer, that was making him so sick. In fact, he had never been sick from cancer.

I found myself thinking, *"What if Bullet was misdiagnosed? What if I'm putting him through treatment—perhaps killing him with it—and he doesn't even have cancer!"* This thought haunted me.

I asked Dr. Porzio and Dr. Hoskins about the possibility of a misdiagnosis. They both assured me that there was no chance of any such thing. They reminded me that the biopsy had been evaluated by two different diagnosticians and that there was no uncertainty about it.

Their certainty saddened me, because it pulled me out of my momentary lapse into denial. But it also forced me to once again face that Bullet really did have lymphoma. Even though it was a disappointment, it reinforced my resolve to keep fighting without worrying that I was making Bullet suffer for no good reason.

I also discussed with Dr. Porzio what would happen "at the end." We agreed on a course of action. The conversation gave me a comforting sense of preparedness and alleviated my anxieties. When I got home, I called the pet crematorium in my area, Hartsdale Pet Cemetery & Crematory. I asked about their hours and what I should do if their services were needed, for example, on a Sunday night. I asked about the cremation procedure and the prices.

If possible, plan for the end when the end is *not* near. Make your decisions about the medical plan and the logistics. This is not a cheery or pleasant task, but having your plans set will alleviate a great deal of anxiety later. Make these decisions

# RESOURCES ON THE NET

There's a wealth of information at your fingertips if you know how to find it. Start by exploring the web sites managed by veterinary schools (see page 25). There you'll find information about research, treatment and clinical trials .

There are many reliable resources on the net. A few are listed below.

### GENERAL INFO WEB SITES
www.vetcancersociety.org
www.cancer.gov
www.perseusfoundation.org/
www.avma.org
www.cvm.tamu.edu/oncology/
www.gcvs.com/oncology
www.vetmed.ucdavis.edu/
www.morrisanimalfoundation.org/

To search further, start with a search engine. Just start plugging in words. It might take you a while and several word combinations before you find what you're looking for—be patient. Use various combinations such as "chemotherapy + dogs," "canine + cancer," or "veterinary + oncology."

At each web site, you'll find links to other sites. Links are usually blue and underlined. Click on any links that look promising or pique your interest. Save good web sites as "bookmarks" or "favorites," or print out important pages during your search. As you branch off from web site to web site and click from link to link, you will eventually and inevitably forget where you started.

You can also use a search engine to research medications and treatments, supplements, clinical trials and diets for canine cancer or for a particular type of canine cancer. If you hear of a supplement that might help your dog, open your search engine and type in its name to search for information about it.

The Internet can be a wonderful resource, but be forewarned: Some information you come across may not be accurate. Check the source and validity of information that you find on the net before adding it to your treatment plan.

### SUPPORT GROUPS ONLINE
Online support groups for people with cancer dogs are invaluable. There's a circular dynamic apparent within these groups: A distraught newcomer posts an urgent plea for help and receives mountains of information and loving support. Before long, the new member has the knowledge and experience needed to become a teacher and supporter of the next rash of new members who are posting urgent pleas for help.

E-groups devoted to pet cancer are listed below. You can participate if you choose to, or read the questions, answers and advice posted by others.

http://forums.delphiforums.com/
  petcancer
http://pets.groups.yahoo.com/group
  /LymphomaHeartDogs
http://pets.groups.yahoo.com/group
  /bonecancerdogs
http://pets.groups.yahoo.com/group
  /CanineCancer
http://groups.yahoo.com/group/
  endlesslove

### THE MAGIC BULLET FUND
If you are able to, please sponsor a dog in treatment. If you have a dog with cancer but cannot afford treatment, apply for help.

www.themagicbulletfund.org

with a clear mind and when the end does come, you will not feel panicky about what will happen. Please don't put this off!

## READ, READ, READ

If you're "On the net," you'll find there a wealth of information on canine cancer. You can access a great deal of information quickly, including current theories about canine cancer treatment and newly discovered cancer-fighting supplements (see "Resources on the Net," page 15). Always double-check the accuracy of information you garner from the Internet with your veterinarian.

Don't forget to listen to your dog! If you watch and listen closely, you will learn about what he wants and what he needs. You may think he's only capable of communicating that he wants to eat or has to pee, but don't discount the possibility that he can tell you much more than that. Watch his facial expressions and body language. Read *Dog Language: An Encyclopedia of Canine Behavior,* by Roger Abrantes. Dogwise Publishing, 2001.

## "IT'S JUST A DOG!"

What *is* a dog's life worth? The typical pet dog will not grow up, develop a career and contribute to society. He will not support you in your senior years or take care of you when you become feeble. He won't even bring you a cup of tea when you've got the flu! (My apologies to Search and Rescue Dogs, Guide Dogs, seizure alert and all other working dogs for this generalization.)

Dogs *will* give unconditional love, loyalty and companionship. Indeed, a dog will devote his entire existence to the solitary purpose of pleasing the special person or persons in his life. This is the gift of the dog. In return, we must at the very least give our dogs love, excellent care and respect.

As cancer-dog caretakers, we are forced to make very difficult decisions about things like surgery, radiation therapy, chemotherapy, palliative care and euthanasia. None of the options are appealing, but we must choose nonetheless. So long as your decisions come from your heart, so long as they are made with love and respect, they are the right decisions.

Are you committed to taking the journey through cancer treatment with your dog? If so, many will understand your decision. People go to great lengths to care for and provide medical treatment for a beloved dog. Some caretakers refinance a home to pay for canine cancer treatment, or take out a bank loan. Some take a leave of absence from work to care for their cancer dogs.

16

And then there are those who simply cannot and will never understand. They say, "But *it's just a dog!*" Don't let these naysayers sway you, but don't think for a moment that you will sway them. At the very most, you'll only convince them that you're entitled to your [nutty] beliefs about the value of a dog's life.

One popular dog book author states that dogs "should not" be treated like human family members. They "should not" be given treatment for cancer. Should we not mend their broken legs either? Where should we draw the line? To me, and surely to most reading this book, our pets *are* family members and they *are* sentient, living beings whose lives *do* have intrinsic value. I apologize for the departure and will get off my "Bully" pulpit right now!

Whether you decide to shore up your resources and marshal your forces to wage war against your dog's cancer, or to release him through early euthanasia to spare him any suffering, make peace with your decision. You will not err if you make this decision with love and respect for your dog as a valuable, sentient creature who is a member of your family who has given you his all and has asked so very little in return.

# Notes

# EARLY DECISIONS

*When choosing a path for your cancer dog,*
*There are no right or wrong decisions.*
*There's no way of knowing what the outcome*
*would have been had you chosen differently.*
*So believe that the decision you've made is for the best.*

When cancer is suspected, the first task is to establish a diagnosis. A veterinarian may be able to establish a preliminary diagnosis of a mass or tumor with some degree of certainty based only on observation and a hands-on examination. A definitive diagnosis, however, is necessary in order for the doctor to formulate a prognosis and determine what type of treatment is appropriate. Seek out a second opinion and an alternate interpretation of test results if there is any possibility of a misdiagnosis.

A diagnosis can be ascertained in several ways. Often, a diagnosis is based on the results of a fine-needle aspirate biopsy. If you can feel the mass with your fingers, a needle biopsy will probably be attempted. A needle biopsy is less invasive, less traumatic and less expensive than a surgical or incisional biopsy. It's is a very simple procedure, generally done without anesthesia. Fluid or tissue cells are extracted from the mass through a needle, and studied under a microscope to determine if there are cancer cells present. The procedure is unsuccessful if fluid from the tumor cannot be extracted.

When a needle biopsy fails to render a diagnosis, an incisional or surgical biopsy is performed. The biopsy report (which you should get a copy of) usually states the type of cancer found, or names the "differentials." The differentials are the best and worst possisble types of cancer that might be present. Of course there is no good type of cancer—this can be stated as the most benign to the most malignant, or the least to most aggressive. Biopsy reports might also estimate the stage of the cancer.

If a surgical biopsy is necessary, please ask your veterinarian to consult a specialist (board certified oncologist or surgeon) before operating. In some cases, it's best to remove the tumor instead of merely taking a tissue sample for diagnostic use. In some cases, it's best to do so with wide margins, to avoid the possible need for a second surgery. Tissue-testing equipment required to achieve "clean margins," is generally found only in the clinic of a board certified veterinary oncologist. A specialist's recommendations are needed.

---

## DECISIONS YOU CAN MAKE

▶ **Consultants:** Choose your team members by referral or reputation and revise at will. It's your team and you must feel that each member is an asset to the team. The goal is to have the strongest team possible. The opposing team is formidable.

▶ **Tests:** You have a great deal of say-so when it comes to testing. You can decline a test based on your dog's comfort level and the benefit to be gained by having the test. Gather information and consult with your team—the final decision is yours.

▶ **Leave or Wait:** If being left at the veterinarian's office is stressful for your dog, wait for the procedure and take him with you whenever possible. Remember, no one wants to be in a hospital longer than necessary—dogs included.

▶ **Shaving:** It's often necessary to shave some fur before surgery or chemotherapy, but generally not for a blood test. It's easier and quicker for the veterinarian to shave but most will, if asked, make the extra effort to draw blood without shaving.

Make every attempt to keep your dog intact and beautiful during treatment. It's easy to wind up with a patchwork dog, so keep the shaving to a minimum from the start.

You can specify which leg should be used for testing and treatment. If, for example, your dog is favoring a leg, you can request that a different leg be used for treatment.

▶ **Revisions:** If your dog isn't able to tolerate a treatment, ask your team members to suggest other options. There may well be another treatment that's equally effective and that your dog can better tolerate. If your dog is very ill, consider postponing the next treatment until he's stronger.

You're not at the mercy of any prescribed treatments, medications or schedules, but stick to the plan unless there's a reason to revise it.

A bone marrow biopsy may be indicated. When a dog has a low white blood cell count (WBC), absolute neutrophils count or red blood cell count (hematocrit), that does not recover quickly, your doctor may want to find out if the bone marrow's ability to produce new blood cells has been compromised by the invasion of cancer cells, or by chemotherapy. A large needle is inserted and "punched" into a bone to remove a sample containing bone cells and marrow cells.

Some tumors require diagnosis via ultrasound, radiography (x-ray) or nuclear scintigraphy (bone scan). Brain and spinal cord tumors are often diagnosed via magnetic resonance imaging (MRI) because they are difficult to access by other methods. Brain surgery is generally too radical and invasive a procedure to perform merely to obtain a diagnosis.

## TREATMENT DECISIONS

When your veterinarian finds that your dog has cancer, he may refer you to a veterinary oncologist—a specialist in veterinary cancer. The specialist will examine your dog, review his medical history and recommend a treatment plan.

When there's no reasonable hope of treatment success, your veterinarian may recommend palliative care (pawspice, or end-of-life care). In palliative care, you do not aim to cure or fight your dog's cancer. You maximize your pet's comfort level and quality of life during the time he has left, and you hope to prolong that period of time.

Your first decision is whether or not to go ahead with treatment. Declining treatment, you can simply enjoy the time you have left with your dog and let nature take its course, but a decision to decline medical treatment does not mean that there's nothing you can do! You can still help your dog fight cancer and be as healthy and happy as possible, and perhaps survive longer.

In an effort to buy some time, slow down the disease process and postpone the decline, use the same dietary and supplemental measures used by those who do provide medical treatment. To read about dietary measures that benefit cancer patients, read Chapter 7. For information about supplements that may improve your dog's quality of life and perhaps prolong his life, read Chapter 8.

If you decide to treat the cancer aggressively, the course of action may be clear. One treatment option may be most effective for the type of cancer that your dog has. But often, there are several treatments and no definitive studies showing which one has the best chance of success.

You can be an active participant in the decision-making process for your dog's treatment without having a degree in veterinary medicine. If you have a limited understanding of medicine but want the best chance of success, consult the experts. Join an online support group and ask the members for input based on their experiences. Then make an informed decision based on all of the recommendations.

Whenever you have reservations about a recommended treatment, seek out a second opinion and even a third, if the first two conflict with each other. Often, a doctor will recommend the treatment or protocol with which he is most familiar. It may or may not be the one that will be most effective for your dog. Some veterinary oncologists at the schools of veterinary medicine and in private practice are willing to answer questions by email or phone to help you decide.

Your veterinarian, and any consultants that you enlist, will help you determine what your options are, depending on the type, stage and grade of cancer, and the overall health of your dog. You have now taken the first step toward assembling a team. *"What team?"* You will launch an attack against your dog's cancer and it will involve a larger cast than just you, your dog and a veterinarian. You are the Captain of that team!

# CHOOSING A DOCTOR

To earn the title "veterinary oncologist," veterinarians must complete at least two or three years of rigorous clinical experience and training and then pass a two-day theoretical and practical examination.

A board certified veterinary oncologist should be included as a member of your team either as your dog's primary cancer treatment provider, or as a consultant. Three factors will help you decide which of these roles the oncologist plays on your team: Proximity (there may not be a veterinary oncologist near you); Cost (a board certified oncologist's fees are typically higher than a general practice veterinarian's); Familiarity (this is important if your dog has fearful or aggressive tendencies and is at ease with his regular doctor).

There are hundreds of thousands of dogs with cancer in the U.S. and only about 200 board certified veterinary oncologists. Obviously, it's just not possible for every cancer dog to be treated by an oncologist. To fill the gap, many veterinarians have become proficient at cancer treatment. You may be able to find a general practice veterinarian, or a resident in oncology who has not yet passed the board exam, to provide cancer treatment for your dog.

# ASSEMBLE YOUR TEAM

The size and scope of your team is entirely up to you—you are the captain of the team! Don't be afraid to add to and redefine your team roster. You should have complete and implicit confidence in each of your practitioners and consultants. Each of your team members must have expert knowledge in the facet of cancer treatment to which they are going to contribute to your dog's treatment or care, and they should be invested in seeing your dog survive with a good quality of life.

▸ **Your veterinarian,** who knows your dog's personality and medical history better than any other member of your team. Some general practice veterinarians provide cancer treatment in addition to running a general practice. They should and usually do each have an oncologist consultant who steps in to offer direction and advice when necessary.

▸ **A board certified veterinary oncologist** at a veterinary school or major veterinary hospital is an essential member of the team. He has access to cutting edge information about new and revised treatment recommendations and experimental treatments not yet in general use. Your oncologist may provide your dog's treatment or may act as a consultant to the veterinarian providing treatment, and be available for consultation when necessary throughout the course of treatment.

The doctor providing treatment, whether a general practice veterinarian or a veterinary oncologist, will provide test results and progress reports to you and also to the other members of your team when appropriate.

▸ **A holistic veterinarian.** Holistic veterinary medicine can enhance and supplement traditional treatments. If you forgo traditional treatment entirely, a holistic veterinarian can serve as your dog's primary doctor.

If your general practice veterinarian is holistic, do enlist an allopathic (traditional) team member so that you can receive input from both camps.

Some holistic veterinarians are "purists" and will refuse to treat your dog if he is undergoing traditional treatment. Likewise, some traditional veterinarians will refuse to treat your dog if you employ certain holistic methods. If you wish to use a combination of holistic and traditional therapies, as I have, you'll need to find open-minded team members.

▸ **Specialists,** as needed, will treat secondary or unrelated health problems that arise. Any team member can refer you to an appropriate specialist. All specialists must be informed of your dog's cancer status and treatment.

▸ **Other caretakers of dogs with cancer:** Your veterinarian may put you in touch with one of his other clients, or you may already know someone fitting this description. Join an online support group! A great deal of information is exchanged among caretakers of cancer dogs online (see "Resources on the Net," page 15).

▸ For dogs with cancer requiring radiation therapy and/or surgery, the caretaker will enlist a board certified radiation oncologist and/or a board certified surgeon, accordingly.

Most general practice veterinarians who treat cancer do so in addition to annual check-ups, emergency procedures, spays and neuters. The veterinary oncologist devotes his full attention to cancer treatment and has far more experience and expertise in treating cancer. Because of the glut of cancer dogs and the shortage of oncologists, many general practice veterinarians provide cancer treatment and have become expert at it.

Once the treatment plan is in place, if treatment goes smoothly the consultant may not be needed at all. However, more often than not, adjustments have to be made, and then our doctor will contact the consultant for assistance. You may at any time ask your doctor to consult a specialist.

Many oncologists at veterinary schools or in private practice provide telephone consultations to veterinarians treating cancer dogs. Sometimes there is a fee. The specialist can advise your veterinarian of the best treatment plan.

If your veterinarian doesn't have a relationship with an oncologist, you may need to enlist one. Contact the veterinary school nearest to you (see page 25) or the American College of Veterinary Internal Medicine [www.acvim.org], or ask for assistance from The Magic Bullet Fund at [www.themagicbulletfund.org/oncologists.html].

Some veterinarians don't have an oncology consultant, but instead take advantage of telemedicine technology. According to Dr. Hoskins,

*Many veterinarians employ telemedicine to get input from specialists when there isn't one on staff. For example, digital X-rays and ultrasound images can be generated on-site and transmitted to a specialist anywhere in the world for interpretation and consultation.*

In November 2002, Bullet developed a heart condition. Electrocardiograms (ECGs) were performed on Bullet in Dr. Hoskins' hospital, where there is no cardiologist on staff. Bullet's ECG was transmitted to Cardiopet while it was being done, while I was kissing his beautiful face. Cardiopet's veterinary cardiologists interpreted the results and faxed a report to the clinic within 24 hours, along with a diagnosis, prognosis and explicit treatment recommendations.

Oncura Partners™, the oncological equivalent of Cardiopet, provides expert consultation and guidance to general practice veterinarians who treat cancer.

To find a holistic veterinarian in your area, visit [www.holisticvetlist.com] or call (410) 569-0795. To find an oncology radiologist, download the file [www.vetcancersociety.org/pdf/radiation.pdf] from the Internet.

# SCHOOLS OF VETERINARY MEDICINE

| SCHOOL | PHONE | WEB SITE |
|---|---|---|
| Auburn University | (334) 844-2685 | www.vetmed.auburn.edu/index.pl/oncology_info |
| University of California-Davis | (530) 752-1393 /0186 | www.vmth.ucdavis.edu/vmth/services/oncology/oncology.html |
| Colorado State University | (970-297-4195 | www.csuanimalcancercenter.org |
| Cornell University | (607) 253-3060 | www.vet.cornell.edu/cancer/referral.html |
| University of Florida | (352) 392-4700 | www.vetmed.ufl.edu/sacs/Oncology/oncology.htm |
| University of Georgia | (706) 542-3461 | www.vetmed.iastate.edu |
| University of Illinois-Urbana | (217) 333-5300 | www.cvm.uiuc.edu/vth/genonco.htmlwww.vetmed.lsu.edu |
| Iowa State University | (515) 294-4900 | www.vetmed.iastate.edu/services/vth/clientinfo |
| Kansas State University | (785) 532-5690 | www.vet.ksu.edu/depts/VMTH/oncology/index.htm |
| Louisiana State University | (225)578-9600 | www.vetmed.lsu.edu/vth&c/oncology.htm |
| Michigan State University | (517) 353-4523 /5420 | www.cvm.msu.edu/vth/cco/index.htm |
| University of Minnesota | (612) 625-1919 | www.cvm.umn.edu/vmc |
| Mississippi State University | (662) 325-1351 /3432 | www.cvm.msstate.edu/ahc/ |
| University of Missouri | (573) 882-7821 /4589 | www.vmth.missouri.edu |
| North Carolina State University | (919) 513-6690 | www.cvm.ncsu.edu/docs/onconcacp.html |
| Ohio State University | (614) 293-7517 | www.vet.ohiostate.edu/ |
| Oklahoma State University | (405) 744-6648 | www.cvm.okstate.edu/ |
| Oregon State University | (541) 737-2858 | www.vet.orst.edu |
| University of Pennsylvania | (215) 898-4680 /4685 | www.vet.upenn.edu/ryan |
| Purdue University | (765) 494-1107 | www.vet.purdue.edu/ |
| University of Tennessee | (865) 974-8387 | www.vet.utk.edu/radiology/oncology |
| Texas A&M University | (979) 845-2351 | www.cvm.tamu.edu/oncology |
| Tufts University | (508) 839-5395 | www.tufts.edu/vet/sah/harrington.html |
| Tuskegee University | (334) 727-8174 | www.tuskegee.edu |
| Virginia-Maryland Regional College of Veterinary Medicine | (540) 231-4621 | www.vth.vt.edu/home.asp |
| Washington State University | (509) 335-0751 /0752 | www.vetmed.wsu.edu/depts-vth/smallAnimalServices.asp |
| Western University | (909) 469-5628 | www.westernu.edu/veterinary/clinic.xml |
| University of Wisconsin-Madison | (608) 263-7600 | vmthpub.vetmed.wisc.edu/sa_services |

# To Test or Not To Test

During the diagnosis stage, your veterinarian most likely did some blood work, either a fine-needle aspirate biopsy or a surgical biopsy, and possibly a bone marrow biopsy. There's no getting around it—initial diagnostics really are necessary. But, from this point on, the caretaker must be discriminating. Discuss with your veterinarian the expected results and potential benefits of any recommended test. Discuss the expected discomfort, pain level or trauma to your dog and the costs to you. If the potential benefits do not outweigh the potential suffering and the expense, "Just say no!"

Anesthetics are poisons. Any test that requires anesthesia should be declined unless the results might contribute significant information about your dog's status that will determine what treatment or medication will be most effective.

At the time of Bullet's first chemotherapy treatment, two tests were suggested. The first was a bone marrow biopsy. There was no reason to believe that he had any type of bone cancer and there was no sign of myelosuppression. I asked what purpose the test would serve, and Dr. Porzio explained that it would give us an idea of how advanced the cancer was. Would the results alter Bullet's treatment plan? *"Not at all."* In other

words, the result of this test would allow the doctor to fine-tune the prognosis, and I would be able to make a note in my date book on the day that Bullet was expected to come out of remission. Because this test can be uncomfortable or painful and because the result was not going to improve our treatment plan at all, *and* because I had no interest in writing that date in my calendar, I declined the bone marrow test.

The second test that Dr. Porzio suggested was an ultrasound on Bullet's heart, that was to be done before using the chemotherapy agent doxorubicin (Adriamycin®). This is a highly cardiotoxic agent that cannot be given if a dog's heart function is not strong enough to tolerate it. It is generally done before every treatment with "adria" and I agreed to this test.

Don't passively agree to all tests, but don't summarily reject all tests either. Gather information and weed out any tests that are not going to benefit your dog. Of the tests that might benefit him, you take on the difficult task of weighing trauma and expense against benefit. Will the test be traumatic for your dog? What are the chances that it will provide information that will alter or fine-tune his treatment plan? To what degree might it benefit him? This is not an easy task, but you will think it through, seek out the advice of your expert team members and make the best decision you can.

## TO TREAT OR NOT TO TREAT

Deciding whether or not to provide treatment for a dog with cancer can be difficult. If you're unable to make the decision, give thought to each factor in "Considerations for Treatment," page 27.

Think through all of the options. Clarify your feelings and thoughts about each and the reasons you can think of to choose or not to choose each. Once you've made a decision, do not second-guess yourself! There's no way to know what the outcome would have been had you chosen differently, so trust and believe that the decision you made was for the best.

If you decide to treat your dog's cancer but treatment isn't successful, will you have made the wrong choice? Of course not. If you don't treat or stop treatment and the cancer returns, don't torture yourself by asking "What If..."

Think about what you would choose if you were in his place. Would you undergo any and all treatments that might grant you another month? Another year? What if the treatment was a painful one?

Whether or not to treat, which treatment to use

and when (if ever) to stop treatment are all difficult decisions. It might help you to decide if you ask your team members the following questions.

QUESTIONS TO ASK YOUR VETERINARIAN

▸ What's the *best* possible outcome (i.e., cure or length of remission) of this treatment? How often is that achieved? What studies or tests were done to find these statistics?

▸ How invasive/traumatic would this treatment be for my dog?

▸ What's the *worst* possible outcome? Is it that the treatment simply won't work, or might my dog have adverse reactions? If so, what are they and what percentage of dogs have these reactions?

▸ If the treatment isn't successful, what is Plan B? (Ask the questions above again, about Plan B.)

▸ What is the total cost of this treatment if it works? If it doesn't work?

▸ What would you do if this was your dog?

## FINANCIAL CONSIDERATIONS

Financial considerations are often a deciding factor, but there are ways to reduce the costs of treatment. Find a pharmacy selling the chemotherapy agents at a discount and ask your veterinarian to provide a prescription. Ask about purchasing chemotherapy agents that are close to their expiration date, or a generation old.

Request that the least expensive protocol be chosen; that dosages be reduced (to 75 percent, for example); that treatments are scheduled less frequently. Dosages and schedules in a protocol are based on what is most effective for most dogs, but the study groups are usually small. Protocols are altered all the time when a dog has adverse effects, or when the cancer doesn't regress. Don't hesitate

---

## CONSIDERATIONS FOR TREATMENT

▸ **The Age and Health of Your Dog.** In a geriatric dog, we must ask if the treatment is painful or traumatic for the dog. If so, how likely is it that after enduring the treatment, the dog's life will be extended appreciably? A dog of any age with preexisting medical issues may not tolerate treatment well, and a preexisting condition may decrease the probability of success. Consider a treatment option that is less traumatic for the dog, even if it has a somewhat lower success rate.

▸ **Quality of Life.** How will treatment affect your dog's quality of life? Weigh the chances of treatment success against the possibility and degree of trauma your dog may endure from the treatment. There are many factors to weigh and there is no right answer except the one that comes from your heart.

▸ **Input from Friends and Family.** Seek advice from people who value the life of a dog as highly as you do—people who will help you make a decision that's comfortable for you and right for your dog.

▸ **Gut Instincts.** Evaluate your dog's stamina and ability to endure medical interventions. If you have a strong suspicion that medical intervention will not be successful, you may choose to forgo treatment. Take your psychological makeup into account as well. Are you prepared to roll up your sleeves, clean up vomit and diarrhea and possibly watch your dog endure periods of illness during treatment?

▸ **Financial Considerations.** Thinking of finances when making this decision is difficult emotionally. Are you putting a price on your dog's life? How much time will $1,000 buy him? How much money is it worth to keep him alive three more months? Two years? If you don't spend the money to keep him alive, will you regret it? If you do and the treatment isn't successful, will you regret having spent the money?

▸ **Be Decisive.** Make a decision that won't result in a haunting voice saying *"I should have"* or *"I shouldn't have."* Make the best decision that you can and then accept, regardless of the outcome, that it was the best decision. If you have health insurance for your dog, great! Calculate the extent of coverage so that there won't be any surprises later. If not, you may want to look into policies for your other pets, remembering that 50 percent of our cats and dogs will have cancer in their lifetimes.

to request a variation of a protocol if it will enable you to provide treatment.

If you don't have a pet insurance policy for your dog, this is a wake up call! Now you understand why it's important to have policies for your pets. It's the difference between being able to provide treatment and not being able to. Please find a pet insurance policy for your other pets and your future pets. You will find a few of the best policies at the web site below.

Seek out organizations that provide financial aid for sick dogs. I founded The Magic Bullet Fund in honor of Bullet. The fund helps people whose dogs would not have treatment without our help.

If you are able to, please donate to the fund to help us help someone else's dog. Donate online at [www.themagicbulletfund.org], or mail a check to The Magic Bullet Fund, PO Box 2574, Briarcliff New York 10510.

# GET A MOVE ON!

Don't deliberate too long! Get your dog's treatment started ASAP and you can iron out the fine points, even switch oncologists or treatment plans, later. Why the urgency? Early detection and prompt treatment are the keys to success. In most cancers, the sooner you begin, the better the prognosis. Many types of cancer grow or spread rapidly if left untreated. All cancers are a threat to normal, healthy functioning.

Without treatment, cancers grow increasingly stronger and more widespread and thus more difficult to treat. Once cancer cells have migrated into the bloodstream, the cancer is said to have *metastasized*. Once metastasis has occurred, a new tumor may develop in a different part of the body. Then, the disease continues to progress and the prognosis worsens considerably.

*Notes*

# About Canine Cancer    3

*Cancer is a ruthless foe*
*Without prejudice or discrimination.*
*It attacks even the innocents that share our lives,*
*The cats and dogs, ferrets and rabbits*
*Who have found their rightful places*
*In our homes and in our hearts.*

In recent years, it seems an epidemic of canine cancer has erupted. Everyone I speak to tells me that their dog or a friend's dog has cancer. Every newspaper or magazine has a story about a dog with cancer. I go to a restaurant with a friend and, invariably, someone at an adjacent table is talking about their dog's cancer treatment or a friend's dog's with cancer or about a dog that just lost the battle against cancer.

At first I thought that this was happening simply because I write about it and administer The Magic Bullet Fund, but no, it was not that.

The current estimate is that there are more than 65 million pet dogs in the United States. Fifty percent of our dogs will have some type of cancer in their lifetimes—a widely accepted estimate in veterinary oncology. Thirty million of the dogs that are now in our homes and our hearts are destined to be diagnosed with cancer.

The Animal Cancer Institute provides another statistic, estimating the number of canine cancer cases diagnosed each year as follows: "Using crude estimates of cancer incidence, there are roughly 4 million new cancer diagnoses in dogs...made each year."[1]

According to a more recent report from PBS, aired on March 15, 2007, "It's estimated that, every year in the United States, 10 percent of all dogs develop some form of cancer." That's more than 6 million dogs, every year!

# TYPES OF CANINE CANCER

The most prevalent canine cancers are the various types of skin cancer (lumps and bumps in or under the skin), occurring at a rate of 450 per 100,000 dogs per year.[2] This means that approximately 274,000 dogs are diagnosed with skin cancer each year. These tumors are often benign (e.g., lipomas) but can be malignant (e.g., mast cell tumors), so a specific diagnosis is necessary to determine the best treatment plan.

A veterinarian or veterinary oncologist may be able to make a preliminary diagnosis by visual examination or palpation. A fine-needle aspirate or surgical biopsy will yield a definitive diagnosis and enable your veterinarian to recommend the best treatment plan.

The second most common canine cancer is mammary cancer. Mammary cancer is the most common malignant tumor in dogs. Mammary tumors occur at a rate of approximately 160 per 100,000 dogs in the population. This means that each year about 97,000 dogs are diagnosed with mammary cancer in the United States.

Of all canine mammary cancer cases, 99 percent are females. The risk of cancer for intact (unspayed) females is 26 percent; for those spayed after the first heat cycle, 8 percent and for those spayed before the first heat, 0.05 percent.[3] In light of these statistics, it is difficult to justify *not* spaying a dog. Please, spay and neuter your pets!

Third in line is lymphosarcoma (lymphoma). Philip Bergman, DVM, MS, PhD, ACVIM at the Bobst Animal Medical Center in New York, NY says, "Lymphoma is the third most common cancer found in dogs, with an incidence of 24 cases per 100,000 dogs per year."[4] Using the American Pet Association's 1999 estimate of dog population, more than 14,600 dogs in the U.S. are diagnosed with lymphoma each year. Another estimate is even more dismal: "A more recent report suggests an overall annual incidence [of canine lymphoma] approaching 110 cases per 100,000 [dogs].[5]

Although lymphoma in humans may be Hodgkin's or Non-Hodgkin's Lymphoma (NHL), canine lymphoma is always the malignant Non-Hodgkin's type. Non-Hodgkin's lymphoma is sometimes abbreviated as LSA (lymphosarcoma).

A statistic from the *Veterinary Medical Database Program* (VMDP) at Purdue University reflects a gradual and consistent increase in the incidence of lymphoma between 1987 and 1997. At the starting point of this study, 0.75 percent of the dogs seen at 20 veterinary institutions had lymphoma. Ten years later, when the study was repeated, 2.0 percent had lymphoma.[6]

# THE MOST COMMON CANINE CANCERS

| Cutaneous Cancers (Skin cancer; "lumps and bumps") | Adenocarcinoma (Mammary Cancer) | Lymphosarcoma (Lymphoma) |
|---|---|---|
| ▸ About 30% of all tumors in dogs are tumors of the skin or subcutaneous tumors. Of these, 70-80% are benign. About 20% of these are Mast Cell Tumors (MCTs). <br> ▸ When possible, MCTs are surgically removed. If cancer cells remain, a second excision or radiation therapy is provided. <br> ▸ If excision isn't possible, radiation therapy is used. About 60% of grade I and II MCTs are cured with radiation therapy alone. <br> ▸ Surgery followed by multi-agent chemotherapy increases treatment success. Single-agent chemotherapy with Prednisone does not. <br> ▸ In metastatic MCT's, cure is rare. Chemotherapy (usually in the form of Prednisone) is commonly used for palliative care. <br> ▸ Melanoma (CMM) is perhaps the most difficult cancer to treat successfully. Research DNA Vaccines now in development and any new treatments or trials you can find. <br> ▸ Breeds Predisposed for Mast Cell Tumors: Mixed breed dogs, Boxers, Boston Terriers, Labrador Retrievers, Beagles, Schnauzers. | ▸ Mammary cancer is rare in male dogs. Of all cancerous tumors in females, 50% are mammary tumors. <br> ▸ Half of all mammary tumors in female dogs are benign. These may become malignant if not removed. <br> ▸ Of malignant mammary tumors, most are adenocarcinomas. The rest are inflammatory carcinomas, sarcomas and carcinosarcomas. <br> ▸ Spaying female dogs before $1^1/_2$ years of age is highly protective against this cancer. <br> ▸ Adenocarcinomas are removed along with any abnormal lymph nodes in the area. <br> ▸ A mastectomy is performed if the tissue outside of the nodule is found to contain cancerous cells. <br> ▸ The prognosis is good if the tumor is self-contained and excised. Prognosis worsens according to the extent that cancer cells have metastasized (spread) or invaded blood or lymphatic vessels. <br> ▸ Breeds Predisposed: Several spaniel breeds, possibly the Poodle and the Dachshund. <br><br> ***Please spay and neuter your pets!*** | ▸ Of all lymphomas in dogs, 80% are multicentric. Average survival is 4 to 6 weeks without chemotherapy. With chemotherapy, 80% achieve remission quickly and a survival time of 12-18 months is common. <br> ▸ Relapses are treated with reinduction or second-line chemotherapy. Each subsequent remission tends to be shorter in duration, often by about half. <br> ▸ Other lymphomas: Mediastinal (the chest cavity—causes coughing, eventually inhibits the dog's ability to breathe); Alimentary (gastrointestinal—causes vomiting, diarrhea, weight loss); Cutaneous and ocular, lymphomas of central nervous system, kidney and bone. <br> ▸ Solitary cutaneous lymphoma tumors may be treated surgically or with radiation therapy, followed by chemotherapy. Diffuse tumors are treated with chemotherapy. <br> ▸ Breeds Predisposed to lymphoma: Golden Retrievers, Cocker Spaniels, Rottweilers, Boxers, Basset Hounds, St. Bernards, Scottish Terriers, Airedale Terriers, English Bulldogs. |

*All statistics are approximate and refer to canine cancers.[7]

# WHY DOGS GET CANCER

Has there been an increase in the incidence of canine cancer? Or does there just seem to have been one? Today's average caretaker is more knowledgeable and diligent about responsible pet care than ever before. Our dogs are living longer, thus giving cancer a larger window of opportunity in which to strike.

Veterinary oncology did not exist as a specialty until the early 1990s, and canine cancer cases were not reported. There were veterinarians who treated cancer, even specialized in it, but without board certification. There may actually *not* be as staggering an increase as it appears.

Advances in diagnostic testing in veterinary medicine have made it possible to diagnose canine cancer earlier and with more clarity. Veterinary cancer treatment is more accessible and more successful than ever before, giving caretakers good reason to pursue a diagnosis.

Most of us have a friend or family member who's had a dog with cancer. As would be expected, the marketplace is flooded with products that claim to help pets fight or survive cancer.

What causes canine cancer—better yet, what causes cancer? There is some good information on the subject but a great deal is still unknown.

Three factors are known to cause canine cancer: Exposure to lawn chemicals causes lymphoma and transitional cell carcinoma of the bladder; Obesity leads to bladder cancer; Second-hand smoke may cause nasal cancer, especially in long-snouted dogs.

### LAWN-CARE PRODUCTS

Lawn-care products, including fertilizers, weed killers (herbicides) and pesticides, are thought to be the number one cause of canine lymphoma. A 2003 study conducted at Purdue University School of Veterinary Medicine concluded the following: "*The risk of transitional cell carcinoma (TCC) was significantly increased among dogs exposed to lawns or gardens treated with both herbicides and insecticides or with herbicides alone.*"[8]

Manufacturers of lawn-care products recommend that pets be kept off of the lawn for 24 hours after application, but this may not be a strong enough warning. The chemicals maybe safe for us, but we don't inhale the powders with our noses an inch from the ground. We don't roll around on and dig in the dirt. Chemicals picked up outdoors on the soles of our shoes or our feet don't end up in our mouths because we don't lick the bottoms of our shoes or feet—at least I don't. But I know that Bullet did and, most likely, your dog does too.

Even if you're careful, the products that your neighbors use on their lawns are easily blown onto your yard by the wind. Despite all of your precautions, your dog can wind up licking those harmful chemicals off of his feet.

Most pesticides that we spray on our bodies are labeled "not for internal use." If you use bug spray on your arm and your dog licks it, he is "using it internally." There are some great alternative non-toxic lawn care ideas in an article titled, "Ten Simple Steps to Ecological Lawn Care."[9] Non-toxic lawn care products are offered by companies such as Home Harvest Garden Supply, Inc.,[10] Peaceful Valley Farm Supply[11] and others.

### HOUSEHOLD CLEANING PRODUCTS

Floor-polishing, carpet-cleaning and oven-cleaning products often contain chemicals that cause cancer (carcinogens). We are a chemical-happy society, but many chemicals that we use are entirely unnecessary. Cleaning a kitchen floor can be accomplished with squeaky-clean results using just hot water and a mild, natural soap. Any stubborn dirt remaining can be cleaned up with an abrasive pad or a stronger cleanser. If you use any cleanser on your floors that you wouldn't eat or drink, be sure to rinse and re-rinse the floors thoroughly after using it.

For in-depth information about safe, non-toxic, home made house-cleaning solutions, visit the web site of Ernestina Parziale, Certified Herbalist: [http://earthnotes.tripod.com/clnrecipes.htm].

### FOOD

If chemicals in the environment cause cancer, what about pesticides used on fruits and vegetables? What about antibiotics and growth hormones injected into food animals and dyes used to make foods more appealing? Can genetically modified food products cause cancer? These questions are equally relevant to the food your dog eats.

Since diet plays a role in the fight against cancer, it may also prevent or cause cancer. In *Food Pets Die For*, author Ann N. Martin says, "Many of the grains used in commercial pet food contain levels of herbicides, pesticides, and fungicides that are cancer-causing agents."[12] Grains that don't pass inspection for use in human foods are often deemed adequate for use in pet foods.

In 2007, melamine was discovered in commercial pet foods, prompting a barrage of pet food recalls. It alarmed me to learn that many pet foods, high quality and low, piggy-back onto lines of mass-produced foods to include "pre-fab" ingredients. Home feeding is a great solution and it's simple to prepare! Please see Chapter 7.

### VACCINES

The administration of annual vaccinations to dogs has been suspected by some veterinarians to be a causative factor in the growing number of canine cancer diagnoses. Vaccinations given to our dogs to protect them from a variety of ills may actually cause cancer. Cancers that develop due to vaccination, from repeated injections at the same site or from adjuvants added to vaccines, are called Vaccinoses or Vaccine Associated Sarcomas. Vaccinosis is more common in cats than in dogs.

In April of 2001, the American Veterinary Medical Association (AVMA) issued the following:

> *... some vaccines provide immunity beyond one year. Revaccination of patients with sufficient immunity does not add measurably to their disease resistance, and may increase their risk of adverse post-vaccination events.*[13]

Holistic and holistically-minded veterinarians are generally against annual vaccinations. Even among traditional veterinarians, the annual vaccine philosophy has fallen out of favor. Veterinarians who still promote annual vaccinations remind us of epidemics that have been avoided or curtailed and about the thousands of canine lives that have been spared by the advent of the vaccine. They vaccinate their own pets. It doesn't make sense, they say, to risk losing a dog to a disease when there's a vaccine that can practically guarantee to safeguard him against it. This makes good sense if there is such a risk, but vaccinating a pet against a disease that is not a threat does not make sense.

An animal with cancer should not receive any vaccines at all. If your dog does not have cancer, you must decide which vaccines you want him to have and which you want to decline. I hope the following list will help you decide. Gather the information through research or by asking your veterinarian.

### CONSIDERATIONS FOR VACCINATION

▸ What are the odds that your pet might contract the disease? What percent of pets in your region have it?

▸ What's the efficacy of the vaccine? To what degree does it protect pets from the disease?

▸ When a pet gets this disease, what is the treatment? Is it successful? Painful? Expensive?

▸ What's the overall prognosis for dogs who contract this disease?

If there's a low incidence of a particular disease in your region, and if the treatment for it is effective and not painful, then the answer is not to vaccinate. At the other end of the spectrum, if there's a significant incidence of the disease in your region and there's no effective, safe and economically viable treatment, then do vaccinate.

In most cases, there's no clear cut-off point at which the incidence is low enough and the treatment success rate is high enough to justify not taking preventive measures. The calculations become even fuzzier when we insert into the equation the question, *"What negative effects might the preventive have on your dog?"*

Weigh the risks of vaccinating against the risks of not vaccinating, research the incidence of the disease in your region and the efficacy of the preventive and then make your best decision.

Whether or not to vaccinate a pet is up to the caretaker, with the exception of the rabies vaccine, required by law in some states unless a waiver is accepted. For information about vaccines and cancer, see pages 106. For a printable vaccine waiver form, see page 132.

### CHEMICALS

The proliferation of chemicals in the environment is an important factor. Chemicals deemed safe for use by humans might harm, kill or cause cancer in a dog. Many products that we use regularly are carried to the ground by gravity after being used. These fumes and residues may not harm us, but we're not inhaling them in a highly concentrated form. A canine's nose and mouth are far closer to the ground than are ours, however, and he may inhale or ingest substances that don't harm us because they make contact with only the soles of our shoes.

Note that the word "non-toxic" on a product label generally means that the product is not harmful to the environment. It does not necessarily mean that it's safe for a dog to breathe, lick off the floor or lick off of his paws. For more information on toxins to dogs, contact the ASPCA's Animal Poison Control Center.

### SPAY AND NEUTER!

One type of cancer in particular can easily be prevented—cancer of the reproductive organs. Mammary cancer and ovarian cancer (females) and testicular cancer (males) can develop only if there are reproductive organs! No ovary = no ovarian cancer. No testicles = no testicular cancer. Give your pet a chance! **Spay and neuter early!**

### PREDISPOSITION BY BREED

Breed is a factor in some canine cancers. Dogs of certain specific breeds are more likely to develop cancer than others.

Certain canine breeds tend to develop certain types of cancer. Here's one example that is very easy to explain. Large and giant breed dogs are more likely to develop osteosarcoma (bone cancer). A 150 pound dog and a 20 pound dog both reach full size in the same approximate 2-year period. One dog's leg bone may grow from three inches long to 18 inches long, in the same amount of time. The accelerated growth of the bones over a short period of time is thought to result in the high incidence of bone cancer that we see in large and giant breeds.

Some types of cancer have become common in a particular breed. Breeders who don't keep medical records for the pups they have sold may continue to breed from a breeding pair that repeatedly produces pups with a high incidence of cancer. Responsible breeders are aware when cancer develops in dogs they produce, and will stop breeding a line that results in cancer, particularly when it is repeatedly the same type of cancer.

For more information about the causes of canine cancer, read *Why Is Cancer Killing Our Pets?* by Deborah Straw.

# MEDICAL INTERVENTIONS 4

*Human oncologists and veterinary oncologists have begun
to collaborate, working toward a common goal.
As a result, there are many promising new treatments
for people and dogs with cancer on the horizon.*

Before cancer treatment can begin, a definitive diagnosis is necessary. Different types of treatment are used for different types of cancer. The type, stage and grade of the cancer are all important factors and with this information, a veterinary oncologist determines which treatment plan will have the best chance of fighting that particular cancer. Chemotherapy, surgery and radiation therapy are the medical interventions most commonly used to fight cancer in dogs (and people as well).

Chemotherapy is the treatment of choice for canine lymphoma. It is also used to cure or manage other types of canine cancer. According to Dr. Porzio, "Many malignancies, including but not limited to lymphoma, have already spread at the time of diagnosis. Hence, the importance of chemotherapy, with or without surgery."

If chemotherapy is agreed upon, a protocol is chosen. Protocols are very clear about drugs, dosages and schedules. See Chapter 5 for more information about chemotherapy and page 57 for more information about protocols

## DIAGNOSTICS

When a veterinarian suspects that a dog has cancer, he palpates the lump or enlarged lymph node and attempts a fine-needle aspirate biopsy. If a diagnosis can't be made using this method, an incisional or surgical biopsy or an ultrasound-guided biopsy is needed, to rule out or diagnose cancer. Here, surgery serves a diagnostic purpose.

If a surgical biopsy is needed, you may have an oncologist or a board certified surgeon perform the biopsy. If not, your veterinarian should consult an oncologist before operating. This is important, here's why. Judging by the appearance of the tumor, a specialist may be able to determine that the tumor will have to be removed. With your prior consent, he might opt for that more extensive procedure rather than a biopsy. In that case, the location of the tumor is a determining factor in a decision to remove the tumor entirely, with wide margins, or remove it with minimal tissue and therefore with "dirty margins." These on-the-spot decisions are better made by a specialist with extensive experience. This is important because it can save a dog from having to endure two surgeries rather than one.

# SURGICAL INTERVENTIONS

When surgery is recommended for a dog with cancer, the surgery serves either a *curative* or a *palliative* role. Curative surgery involves the removal of a tumor or a lymph node in an attempt to remove the cancer.

When a cure is the goal, every effort is made to remove the entire tumor as well as surrounding tissue that may contain stray cancer cells. This is called "with wide margins," and it is done in an attempt to achieve "clean margins."

According to Dr. Porzio, "Curative surgery involving the removal of a cancerous [malignant] tumor is generally followed by chemotherapy in order to eradicate stray cancer cells that may remain." Post-surgery chemotherapy is much more important when the margins, according to the biopsy report, are dirty than it is when they are clean.

All of the treatments and procedures that your veterinarian offers are optional. If you are unsure that your pet can tolerate extensive treatment because of his age or general health, you might choose to have the surgery but not the chemotherapy. If the surgery is successful, there may not be cancer cells remaining, in which case chemotherapy is not warranted. Taking into consideration your pet's quality of life, there are sometimes good reasons *not* to do "everything."

Palliative surgical measures are not intended to cure, but instead to reduce pain and/or improve a dog's mobility and quality of life while the cancer runs its course. The incomplete removal of a tumor is a common example of palliative surgery.

Debulking (cytoreductive surgery) of a large tumor may simply make a dog more comfortable. The trauma of major surgery is avoided while improving the quality of life and perhaps prolonging life too.

Surgery is helpful for many types of cancer, including mast cell cancer, melanoma, mammary cancer, hemangiosarcoma and osteosarcoma and various tumors. All tumors should be tested with fine needle aspirate, a very simple procedure that does not require anesthesia.

A malignant tumor that is cutaneous (in the skin) or sub-cutaneous (under the skin) should be removed if possible. Post-surgery success rates (no recurrence of the tumors and no new tumors) vary according to the type, stage and grade of the tumors, the number of tumors and their locations.

Many types of cancer metastasize to the lungs. X-rays are taken before surgery, so that if "lung mets" are found, the caretaker may decide against surgery. When a dog has a short time left, we do not want him to spend his remaining time recovering from surgery! Surgery may proceed despite lung mets if the primary tumor is painful, or if only minor surgery is needed and will benefit the dog's quality of life for his last weeks or months. Once cancer has metastasized to the lungs, there is little to do and palliative care begins.

Osteosarcoma (bone cancer) may be the most difficult type of canine cancer—difficult for the caretaker at the decision making stage. This cancer occurs predominantly in large or giant breed dogs, due to accelerated bone growth. It often appears at a site where there was a previous break, fracture or other damage to the bone.

When the tumor is in a leg, which it most often is, the standard treatment is amputation or leg-sparing surgery, followed by chemotherapy. But bone cancer spreads very quickly to the lungs. By the time diagnosis and amputation have been accomplished, the cancer has already metastasized to the lungs in about 90% of the dogs. At early stages, tumors in the lungs are so small that they are undetectable by current testing methods. These are called "micro-mets" (microscopic metastases). X-ray studies of the lungs are done before a recommendation to amputate. If chemotherapy is given, periodic x-rays are taken to justify continuing treatment.

Caretakers hoping to cure osteosarcoma in their dog amputate as early as possible and pray that the cancer cells have not yet migrated to the lungs. Amputation may be followed up with a chemotherapy protocol to eradicate stray cancer cells. Average survival time is six months to a year. This is about the same as the survival rate with no

# KNOWLEDGE IS POWER

*by Dr. Philip J. Bergman*

I'm happy to have this opportunity to be a part of a book that will help so many pets and the people that love them. You are very likely reading this because your pet has been diagnosed with cancer. That word can be a very frightening one, but be assured that the care of veterinary cancer patients has improved dramatically over the last 20 to 30 years.

Information and education will empower you to make the best decisions for your pet. This can come from a variety of sources, including web sites and newsgroups on the Internet, via personal contacts and via your veterinarian. Information provided in this book will help you to find all of these resources. The best information can be obtained from a veterinary medical oncologist, who will assess your pet and tell you the diagnostic and treatment options. The specialist locator at www.acvim.org will help you locate a veterinary oncologist.

One question that I'm often asked by pet owners is what they can do at home for their pet with cancer. First, love your pet no differently than you normally would. They don't know they have cancer and they therefore do not suffer the psychological implications of the diagnosis as we do.

If you make changes at home (e.g. diet, surroundings and daily routines), do so slowly, one thing at a time. The stress that develops from having to adjust to too many changes at once can actually make a dog or cat sick. It can become difficult to differentiate between the effects of a progression of the cancer vs. changes in the home.

In my work, I have developed a strong interest in immunology as it relates to the treatment and, potentially, prevention of cancer in pets. These areas are so rapidly evolving that, in my opinion, immunotherapy will become a standardized treatment option for pets with cancer in the next 5 to 10 years, with licensed products for veterinary use becoming available within 3 to 5 years.

I'm proud to share with you that, in June of 2007, the melanoma vaccine that I worked on with collaborators at Memorial Sloan-Kettering Cancer Center was given conditional licensure by the USDA. We worked on this vaccine together for 6 years with complete dedication from myself and many medical doctors and veterinar-

ians at MSKCC and AMC. This represents the first vaccine for the treatment of cancer to be approved by the U.S. government. I hope that in the near future, this vaccine will receive full licensure, along with other cancer vaccines soon to be in clinical trials within the BrightHeart network.

BrightHeart Veterinary Centers is a new national network of advanced-care veterinary facilities that works closely with referring veterinarians to provide the highest standards for pet care, to give pets the best chance for longer, healthier lives. You can find more information about BrightHeart at [www.brightheartvet.com].

My heart goes out to you, your family and your pet. What you and your pet are about to go through is a war, and it's a war worth fighting. With the help of a good team including you, your veterinarian, your veterinary oncologist and a great support team, your pet has the best chance for a good quality life.

*Philip J. Bergman DVM, PhD, Diplomate ACVIM (Oncology), Chief Medical Officer (BrightHeart Veterinary Centers, Armonk, NY), Adjunct Associate Faculty Member at Memorial Sloan-Kettering Cancer Center.*

treatment. These treatments are provided with very cautious optimism, and a very hopeful attempt to beat the odds.

In those lucky few, when amputation occurs before the cancer has begun metastasize, the cancer can be eradicated and the dog can have a normal, healthy life on three legs. Yes, "normal"!

If you think that life for a three-legged dog (a tripod) is hard or unhappy or not normal, don't tell the dogs that! Most of them adapt very easily, without skipping a beat. To the amazement of caretakers, most dogs resume all of their normal activities very quickly.

Magic Bullet Fund dog Sophie had chondrosarcoma (a cancer of the tissues outside of the bone). Sophie's right front leg was amputated and no other treatment was provided. This cancer can metastasize but is not as aggressive or as likely to metastasize as is osteosarcoma. Now, 10 months later, Sophie is going strong at 3 years old. We hope she'll have a long, healthy life free of cancer.

Most of the dogs we help in The Magic Bullet Fund are seniors. We strive to achieve additional time with quality of life. But, occasionally, we have the wonderful opportunity to help a young dog with a cancer that can be eradicated and create a true success story. We hope Sophie will have a long, healthy, cancer-free life because of the assistance of The Magic Bullet Fund and those who donated toward her treatment costs.

In the face of osteosarcoma or any bone cancer, some caretakers opt for surgery (most often amputation) followed by chemo; some choose surgery only; others do not provide treatment at all. It's an exceedingly difficult decision that each person must make according to their personal knowledge of what's best for them and their dog.

## RADIATION THERAPY

Radiation treatments are given to dogs with cancer after surgery, along with chemotherapy or as the only treatment modality. Periodically, for several weeks or more, the tumored area is exposed to carefully controlled doses of radiation.

The choice of which therapy/therapies to provide depends on the type, stage and location of the tumor. Radiation therapy is most often the treatment of choice for cancer in the nasal passages and oral cavity, and to treat tumors in the extremities.

Radiation therapy is sometimes given to a dog with cancer in a leg (including bone cancer) after surgery or without surgery, as an alternative for caretakers who are not willing or able to opt for amputation. Radiation therapy is generally a more expensive option.

Half Body Irradiation (HBI) has been used for dogs with lymphoma. Dr. Ruslander reports that this is used at NCSU but adds that no final conclusion has been drawn on the success of this treatment modality. In Dr. Ruslander's words, "The jury's still out about HBI."

Radiation therapy is not without side effects. In *Pets Living With Cancer*, author Robin Downing, DVM, discusses common side effects including desquamation of the skin around any radiated area (an irritation with the appearance of a sunburn), and common effects when radiation is applied to the head. These are faucitis mucositis (an inflammation of the tissue lining the mouth) and dry eye (irritation of tissue around the eyes with decreased tear production).

A Magic Bullet Fund dog called Nakkai had surgery to remove a nerve sheath tumor in her leg. The margins were "dirty," as discovered in the biopsy when cancer cells were detected in the outermost tissue of the biopsy sample. Dirty margins are common when leg tumors are surgically removed, because there is little tissue between the tumor and the bone and this makes it difficult or impossible for the surgeon to take wide margins.

Nakkai's caretaker agreed to have radiation therapy for Nakkai but wanted to use a less aggressive and less damaging protocol than the on

that the radiation oncologist recommended. The doctor refused to give an abbreviated protocol. I negotiated and Nakkai did receive a shortened protocol (less overall treatments) on a looser schedule (three days a week rather than five).

Nakkai had minimal side effects, other than a radiation burn at the surgery site. The open sore that resulted healed in about a month, but the skin is still black and the hair did not grow back. Sharon purchases jazzy sports wristbands to keep Nakkai's bare spot protected. Nakkai was diagnosed in June 2007 and is still going strong in February 2008.

## THERAPIES IN THE PIPELINE

Shortly after Bullet's diagnosis, a veterinarian recommended a certain alternative cancer treatment. I read the literature and asked Dr. Hoskins and Dr. Porzio to read it as well. After hearing their thoughts, I decided against this therapy, even though it just might, some day, turn out to be the "Magic Bullet" against canine lymphoma.

The list of therapies and supplements available is endless, and selectivity is necessary. Choose alternative therapies based on research, test results, empirical data, advice from your team members, and based on your own instincts.

Many new treatments are in development to fight cancer. They are at various stages in the research and development process. Some are being studied in Petri dishes in laboratories at schools of veterinary medicine, while others are farther along in the process and are being used to treat cancer dogs in clinical trials.

All of these new therapies have the potential to become effective in the fight against canine cancer. Many have yet to be tested for safety and consistency and fine-tuned. Trials help to establish the big picture and then the details of precisely how a tool can be used most effectively. Keep in mind that the further along the therapy is in the development process, the more realistically you can hope that it will be effective for your dog.

### CRYOSURGERY

"In the Pipeline" isn't the perfect heading for cryosurgery. This method of treating tumors has found its place with the holistic veterinary practitioner. The treatment is often used for tumors on the skin, eyelid and perianal area and for oral tumors. In cryosurgery, liquid nitrogen or nitrous oxide is used to "freeze" the tumor rather than surgically excising it. Tumor sites that should not be treated with cryosurgery include osteosarcoma of long bones, intranasal tumors, circumferential

anus, large mast cell tumors and other large, aggressive tumors.

Relative to traditional surgery, cryosurgery is a shorter procedure with less trauma to the dog, doesn't require anesthesia and is less costly. If a biopsy is desired, the tissue sample is removed before treatment. When cryosurgery is used, it can't be determined whether or not "clean margins" have been achieved. If your dog has a tumor and cryosurgery is a treatment option, consult a veterinary oncologist before choosing this option.[1]

### HYPERTHERMIA

In a way, hyperthermia is the opposite of cryotherapy. The temperature of tumor cells is raised by ultrasound, microwaves or radiofrequency electrocautery. This treatment hasn't had positive results, but may someday play a role in the fight against cancer, in combination with radiation therapy or chemotherapy. Dr. J. Paul Woods writes, "Hyperthermia offers potential benefit to pets with recurrent, progressive, resistant cancer not amenable to standard therapies."[2]

### PHOTODYNAMIC THERAPY (PDT)

Like cryotherapy and hyperthermia, this treatment exposes cancer cells to a stimulus in hopes that they will, as a result, become damaged (cytotoxicity) and die (necrosis). The goal of these treatment methods—and the goal of most tumor treatment—is to destroy tumor tissue but not the surrounding normal tissues.

In Photodynamic Therapy, the stimulus is a three-way combination including a photosensitizer (IV or topically) to make the tissue more responsive to the treatment a light source and oxygen, which is required to complete the photochemical oxidative process.

PDT is used in veterinary medicine, according to Dr. Dudley McCaw, DVM, diplomate ACVIM, for transitional cell carcinoma and canine oral squamous cell carcinoma. In some countries, it has been approved for use in humans for lung, esophageal, bladder and gastric cancers.[3]

There's a potential for PDT treatment to benefit cancer patients in the future. Much is still unknown about exactly how it works and how to make it work more efficiently.

### IMMUNOTHERAPY

Perhaps the most fascinating studies are those that explore the viability of fighting and/or curing cancer through immunotherapy. This is a very complex and fascinating technology that is showing promising signs of success. One treatment in this category is monoclonal antibody therapy.

Monoclonal antibody (mab) therapy has made substantial contributions to the fight against cancer in recent years. In a process called xenomouse technology, mice are stimulated to produce large amounts of antibodies—not just any antibodies, but the specific antibodies that are produced to fight a specific cancer cell in a specific species.

Monoclonal antibodies are therefore disease-specific and species-specific. This means that the mab for one type of canine cancer is different from the mab for another type of canine cancer (disease-specific) and the mab for a certain cancer in canines is different from the mab for that same cancer in humans (species-specific).

Once produced, the antibodies are extracted from the mouse and delivered to the cancer patient intravenously. Mabs are "targeted therapies," because they affect very specific cancer cells and do not harm healthy cells. Traditional chemotherapy is not targeted, because it acts on all cells in a certain stage of cell division, including healthy cells as well as cancer cells.

Three mabs, Rituxan®, Zevalin® and Bexxar®, have been approved for use in fighting Non-Hodgkin's Lymphoma in humans. Herceptin® (trastuzumab) is a mab that combats breast cancer in humans. These are available and in common use today.

The monoclonal antibody developed to fight canine lymphoma was called mab-231. Mab-231 was available shortly before Bullet's diagnosis. It was used along with chemotherapy, not instead. I was interested to learn more about mab-231 and searched for information about it. I contacted the laboratory that developed it and the distributor, but people I spoke to said that it has vanished, possibly due to a lack of demand.

### VACCINE THERAPY

Dr. Bergman is involved in research and development of vaccine therapy for canine malignant melanoma. Dr. Bergman says:

*Canine malignant melanoma (CMM) is an aggressive cancer that commonly spreads and is resistant to standardized therapies. Novel therapies are desperately needed for this extremely malignant tumor. At present, standardized therapies generally translates to median survival times (MST) of 3 to 6 months for dogs with advanced CMM. However, the MST for dogs with advanced CMM treated with surgery or radiation followed by DNA vaccine is approaching 2 years.*

Magic Bullet Fund dog Kirby came to the fund with oral melanoma. Kirby's caretaker, Blake, researched canine melanoma and found informa-tion about a vaccine in development for the treatment of canine melanoma. It was the same DNA vaccine that Dr. Bergman mentioned above. Blake brought the information to Dr. Alice Villalobos at the VCA in Hermosa Beach, CA., and the doctor made arrangements to give Kirby treatment with Merial's DNA vaccine for CMM, which was being used under conditional licensing from the FDA.

Kirby has not developed new CMM tumors, but eight months after treatment began, an x-ray revealed nodules in her lungs. In general, once there are "lung mets," treatment is terminated. However, Dr. Bergman provided information indicating that in addition to fighting CMM, the vaccine may actually slow the progression of secondary lung cancer (cancer metastasized to the lungs). We continue to provide Kirby with DNA vaccine treatments, hoping that the mets will diminish or even vanish.

### ANTIANGIOGENESIS THERAPY

Angio (blood or lymph vessel) genesis (birth) is the development of new blood vessels. Tumors release chemicals that stimulate the production of a new network of blood vessels around the tumor. Without the blood supply provided by a specific type of vessel, tumors are unable to grow. In *Anti*angiogenic therapy, substances that selectively inhibit the generation of these new vessels are introduced in an attempt to cut off a tumor's blood supply and thereby kill the tumor.

Chand Khanna DVM, PhD, diplomate ACVIM (oncology), President of the Animal Cancer Institute and Chairman of the Perseus Foundation, is involved in research using antiangiogenic agents. Dr. Khanna explains this treatment as follows:

> *Agents that inhibit new blood vessel formation or specifically target tumor-associated blood vessels represent a novel, potentially effective and non-toxic treatment for cancer. It is likely that these agents will provide the next major breakthrough in the management of pet animals and people with cancer....*[4]

One antiangiogenesis success story involves a dog called Navy. As of July 2002, Navy had maintained a 16-month remission from lymphoma. This "cure" has not been repeated successfully in any other dogs, but it did inspire new research into antiangiogenesis.[5]

Stories of spontaneous remissions and miracle cures are plentiful. They always lead to a flurry of excitement and a bonanza in sales of the supplements that were given to the dog. It's possible that when spontaneous remission occurs, a random combination of therapies or a genetic anomaly is responsible. It's possible that each cancer requires a different combination of treatments and/or supplements. Occasionally, even a blind squirrel finds an acorn!

# CLINICAL TRIALS

New clinical trials in veterinary oncology are announced on an ongoing basis. Most aim to compare the success rate of an accepted protocol with its success rate when given over an abbreviated or extended time period, in different amounts, dosages, titration, combinations and/or on a different schedule. There are also clinical trials that test the efficacy of a new type of cancer treatment.

The announcement of a clinical trial states that the trial is in progress, explains the procedure and specifies the requirements for enrollment. Most trials have strict requirements for enrollment. Some specify that only dogs who have not undergone chemotherapy and/or radiation therapy may participate; some accept dogs in a certain age range. Some are open only to dogs who are in a first remission; others only to dogs who have relapsed (have come out of remission) several times.

During a clinical trial, participants (dogs with cancer) are monitored closely to document side effects, general health and survival time. In some trials, particularly those using an experimental drug, funding is available to help caretakers manage the costs. Participants may be required to forgo other treatments that have documented success or to grant permission for an autopsy to be performed on the dog if he dies during the trial. Some of the dogs in a trial may receive placebo rather than treatment.

A clinical trial may reveal a new, successful treatment that will not only help your dog but also many other dogs—and, eventually, people—with cancer. Conversely, a clinical trial may prove to be less effective than traditional treatments. When no traditional treatment with a high success rate is available, however, or when budgetary constraints preclude other treatment, enrollment in a clinical trial can be an attractive option.

To learn about clinical trials in which your dog may participate, first ask your veterinarian or veterinary oncologist. If you discover a trial on your own that is appropriate for your dog, ask your veterinarian to become a medical participant in the trial and provide the treatment for your dog.

Clinical trials are routinely conducted at schools of veterinary medicine (see page 25), at large veterinary hospitals with specialty services and at veterinary practices that participate in networks or collaborate with local hospitals.

# COMPARATIVE ONCOLOGY

This recently developed scientific discipline impacts all of us who are involved in any aspect of veterinary oncology. It impacts the caretakers of dogs with cancer, even if most have never even heard of it.

*Comparative Oncology is the study of cancer across species.* Veterinary oncologists and human oncologists work together to study and compare the behavior of cancer in dogs to the behavior of cancer in humans. The goal is to develop successful treatments against cancer in both species.

Dogs and people get the same types of cancer, with few exceptions. Treatment provided to dogs with cancer are the same or only marginally different from treatment provided to people with cancer (and generally less aggressive). There are many parallels to be found when comparing canine cancer to human cancer, but there is one very important difference.

You have probably heard the ballpark estimation that dogs age seven times faster than humans. Well, cancer in the dog also progresses approximately seven times more quickly than it does in the human. A dog's response to therapies and treatments also occurs seven times faster than a human's, and this is of great importance and of great use to scientific researchers, treatment specialists and pharmaceutical companies. Dr. Susan Lana, DVM, DACVIM (oncology) at the Animal Cancer Center at Colorado State University in Fort Collins, CO, says "We're helping the animal patient, but we're also answering some of these preliminary questions into how these medicines or these treatments might translate into human care."

By studying the effects of a cancer treatment in dogs, researchers can evaluate the success rates of a new drug in months rather than years. They can study a new treatment in an accelerated model (the dog) and determine the potential success of that treatment in humans, in 7 months rather than the 4 years it would require too complete the same study in humans.

In Dr. Phil Bergman's contribution to this book on page 42, you will see the following included in his credits at the end of the article: "Adjunct Associate Faculty Member at Memorial Sloan-Kettering Cancer Center." Dr. Bergman earned this title through his work in cooperation with the medical oncologists at Sloan Kettering, in New York City. Dr. Jedd D. Wolchock, MD, PhD, at Sloan-Kettering says about his work with Dr. Bergman, "I saw the opportunity to possibly, in my wildest dreams, help his dogs, but also get some early evidence for safety and efficacy of our vaccine."[6]

The result of this collaborative effort that spans species is the DNA Vaccine for melanoma, now available for use in dogs with melanoma with conditional licensure.

This vaccine is expected to begin FDA Phase II testing soon, on its way to helping people with melanoma. If it does someday lead to treatment that helps people with this deadly cancer, we will owe a debt of gratitude to all those who not only allowed the vaccine to be used on their dogs, but also paid the treatment fees (i.e. development costs) when it was not yet ready for use on humans. Cutting edge research for pet *and human* cancer treatments are regularly tested and financed by loving caretakers like you who are only trying the save their dogs' lives.

# EARLY DETECTION

Early detection is no less important in canine cancer than it is in human cancer. How can cancer in a dog be detected early? See the top 10 signs of cancer in pets, on page 54 of this book. Also find a more comprehensive listing on page 137.

As public awareness about the threat of cancer to dogs increases, so does the desire of caretakers to safeguard, to check and to be informed. The key to finding cancer early, to give your dog the best chance of survival, is to be very observant of his appearance and behavior. When walking your dog, don't talk to a friend or chat on your cell phone! Walk your dog! Pay attention to him, notice if he is limping, panting more than usual, if his stools are not their usual color or consistency. At home, notice his eating and drinking habits so you will know if anything changes.

Annual exams are important! If you do not give your pet vaccines, then ask your veterinarian to do titer tests annually instead. Even if your dog does not have annual vaccines, the annual checkup is still necessary! Allow your veterinarian to draw your dog's blood for a CBC, and to collect or extract urine for urinalysis. Allow your veterinarian to check your dog's teeth and gums, feel for lumps and bumps, etc. A check up once a year for your pet is about equal to a check up once every 7 years for you!

A new blood test to detect early lymphoma in dogs is available to your veterinarian now from Pet-Screen, a U.K. based company. Pet-Screen has several other tests in development to diagnose other types of cancer. The Magic Bullet Fund is helping by sending Pet-Screen blood samples from three dogs in the fund who, unfortunately, have developed lung metastases.

The Lymphoma Blood Test from Pet-Screen detects early canine lymphoma with 84% accuracy. The test may soon be part of every dog's annual exam, particularly dogs at risk due to breed or exposure to carcinogens . The cost varies but may be worth the expense, at about $160.00.

For dogs with lymphoma, Pet-Screen's Directed Chemotherapy Assay takes the guesswork out of a treatment plan. Various chemo agents are applied to a tissue sample to determine which agents do the most damage to the cancer cells. With this information, Pet-Screen recommends the best protocol for that dog and for that cancer. Advanced diagnostics such as these will help caretakers treat canine cancer more successfully.

Read more about canine cancer tests in development on the net at [www.pet-screen.com].

*Notes*

# CHEMOTHERAPY 5

*Treatment can be hard for some but,*
*When it's the only chance for survival,*
*Keep the Faith and say*

**Not Today and Not Without a Fight!**

Cancer may be the "C word" that makes us cringe most, but Chemotherapy is at least a close runner up. Chemotherapy is used to treat various types of cancer in dogs, including lymphoma, acute lymphoid leukemia, chronic lymphocytic leukemia, acute and chronic myelogenous leukemia, multiple myeloma, systemic mast cell tumors, soft-tissue sarcomas, osteosarcoma and carcinomas.[1]

Chemotherapy protocols designed for dogs are less rigorous than are those designed for humans. While many people are willing to undergo extreme, potentially life-threatening treatment in order to have a chance at beating cancer, most pet caretakers are not willing to see their dogs die or become severely ill from treatment. A protocol that is highly toxic can be expected to fall out of favor, even if it has also been found to be highly successful in some cases. Dr. Hahn explains:

*Dogs tend to tolerate chemotherapy better than people do. This is because veterinarians rarely administer maximum dosages—those that would be most aggressive against cancer but would also guarantee severe side effects. Rather, we give dosages that will make only about 10 percent of pets have side effects. Survival times and remission times reported are based upon these "kinder, gentler" dosages. Consult with your veterinary team about your goals and expectations of chemotherapy when your pet is treated.*

# Early Detection of Cancer or of Relapse

### *by Dr. Rodney Page*

Early detection is key to the successful treatment of canine cancer. All dog owners should watch for the early signs of cancer that are listed in the "Ten Common Signs of Cancer in Small Animals" and report any and all findings to their veterinarian.

These signs may also indicate that a dog in remission with cancer has relapsed or developed new cancer sites. In many instances, the need for a second remission does not mean that treatment can no longer provide additional quality time.

I recommend that all dog owners examine their dogs monthly according to the following list. Owners of dogs that have been diagnosed with cancer should conduct the same examination weekly.

---

### Ten Common Signs of Cancer in Small Animals

▸ Abnormal swellings that persist or continue to grow

▸ Sores that do not heal

▸ Weight loss

▸ Loss of appetite

▸ Bleeding or discharge from any body opening

▸ Offensive odor

▸ Difficulty eating or swallowing

▸ Hesitation to exercise or loss of stamina

▸ Persistent lameness or stiffness

▸ Difficulty breathing, urinating or defecating

*Provided by the American Veterinary Medical Association (AVMA)*

\* See page 137 for a more complete list.

---

1. Feel your dog's lymph node regions. See page 13 for a map of the locations of the major lymph nodes on a dog or ask your veterinarian to show you where the nodes are on your dog. Make a note of the size of each node—a mental note and also a notation in your log book for later reference.

2. Feel the mammary glands on female dogs to detect any changes.

3. Go over the skin of your dog's entire body. Make "dermal maps" of any existing lumps and bumps. This will later help you determine how quickly a benign skin bump may be changing.

4. Try to examine the inside of your dog's mouth. This is sometimes challenging but is often easier than expected, depending on the dog's disposition.

5. Annual blood and urine tests are adequate unless there are any abnormalities. Then, schedule rechecks every 4 to 6 months to follow those abnormal results.

6. Twice a year, if possible, your dog should have chest X-rays and abdominal ultrasound, particularly in breeds that are predisposed to splenic hemangiosarcoma (Golden Retrievers and German Shepherd dogs). Although this may sound excessive, remember that dogs age much faster than do humans. An annual visit to the veterinarian is simply not sufficient to protect a geriatric dog.

---

*Rodney Page, DVM, diplomate ACVIM (Internal Medicine, Oncology) is a professor and the director of the Sprecher Institute for Comparative Cancer Research at the College of Veterinary Medicine, Cornell University.*

Lymphoma is said to be the most aggressive form of canine cancer. Most experts—including most holistic veterinarians who are generally opposed to the use of chemotherapy for treating cancer—agree that dogs diagnosed with lymphoma have a life expectancy of only a few weeks without chemotherapy.

Lymphoma is also said to be highly treatable. According to Susan M. Cotter DVM, diplomate ACVIM (Internal Medicine/Oncology), Tufts University School of Veterinary Medicine, with chemotherapy, "Dogs with lymphoma have an average survival of around a year past diagnosis with a good quality of life."

Dr. Ruslander says that of dogs with lymphoma given chemotherapy, approximately 5 to 10 percent achieve a cure. I asked what constitutes a "cure," knowing that the disease is "terminal." Dr. Ruslander responded, "There is a cure when the tumors do not return." (Enlarged lymph nodes are considered to be tumors.)

I asked Kevin A. Hahn, DVM, PhD, diplomate ACVIM (Oncology) the same question and he provided an answer that made more sense to me. Dr. Hahn said:

*It's difficult to say that a dog with lymphoma is "cured," because you never stop looking for new tumors.*

According to Dr. Cotter, lymphoma and leukemia are considered to be systemic from the beginning.

*Like most cancers, these cancers begin as a single cell. However, because these cells are abnormal variants of blood cells, and can thus easily travel through the blood or lymphatic system, the diseases seem to start in many places or in the lymph nodes all at once.*

Until remission is achieved, active cancer cells are busily damaging the body's vital organs including the kidney, spleen, lungs and liver. Many of the cancer-fighting agents used in chemotherapy can themselves cause damage to these organs and to the heart. Once the damage is done, the dog, caretaker and veterinarian are left with not only the cancer to combat, but organ damage or dysfunction as well.

Dr. Cotter says, "A dog that is asymptomatic (i.e., only has enlarged lymph nodes) has a better chance of remission than a dog that has other symptomology related to cancer." The healthier the organs are at the start of chemotherapy, the better able your dog will be to tolerate the internal maelstrom that is created by chemotherapy.

According to Dr. Ruslander, in the case of lymphoma, the stage of the disease does not necessarily determine the potential success of treatment "...unless there's stage V (five) extranodal or bone marrow involvement."

Dr. Porzio agrees, adding that the outcome of chemotherapy treatment for lymphoma appears to be the same regardless of when it begins, so long as there's no organ involvement (no signs that cancer cells are present in an organ, and so long as, at the time cancer treatment begins, the dog has not been previously treated with Prednisone alone. The prognosis is best when a dog is asymptomatic when treatment begins, aside from having enlarged lymph nodes.

Drugs in the corticosteroid family (such as Prednisone), when given alone, can induce a phenomenon called "multidrug resistance."

> *Prednisone used as a single agent may induce drug resistance...If an owner opts to try Prednisone alone first and asks for combination therapy later, the results may not be as good as usually expected.*[2]

Of dogs with lymphoma who have chemotherapy, 80-90 percent achieve remission within the first few treatments—often with a single treatment. The duration of the remission varies greatly, but generally lasts between 3 and 18 months. Then, chemo begins anew in an attempt to achieve a second remission.

With a diagnosis of cancer, we'd all prefer to hear "early stage," but whenever the disease is discovered is the time that you begin. Since it isn't possible to go back in time and discover it at an earlier stage, do what you can now. According to the pathologist's report on Bullet's biopsy, the lymphoma was "late stage." Nonetheless, the first chemotherapy treatment achieved a remission that lasted the rest of his natural life.

## CHEMOTHERAPY SIMPLIFIED

Simply stated, chemotherapy is the application of one or more "agents" designed to kill cancer cells, or at least hinder their ability to multiply and invade healthy cells and progress. Most treatments take less than an hour, but the duration depends on which agent is being administered and also on how cooperative the dog is on that day. The duration also varies depending on the size of the dog. The larger the dog, the greater the volume of chemotherapy agents given, the longer the duration of treatment.

Some agents are administered intravenously, others are injected subcutaneously and others are given orally in pill form. Most of the agents attack cells that are dividing, but some attack at a different stage of cell division than others. And some

# ABOUT PROTOCOLS

A protocol is an attack plan of sorts. It specifies the agents (drugs) that will be given, the dosages and the schedule by which they will be given, week by week, from beginning to end. The choice of a protocol is a strategic decision, similar to deciding whether to deploy the marines, the air force or the navy to attack an enemy.

There are single agent protocols, which use one agent repeatedly until the patient comes out of remission, and combination protocols. The combination protocols are favored for most types of cancer.

Each chemotherapy agent attacks cancer in a different way (i.e., at a different stage during the replication of the cancer cell). Agents are rotated according to a schedule in an attempt to "hit" the cancer with one, then another, then another, hoping for a better shot at killing as many cancer cells as possible (or at least giving them a TKO or a concussion).

Each protocol is unique in which agents it includes, in what order and on what schedule. Many protocol names are composed of the first letters of the agents employed. Because there's a limited number of agents available, similarities between proto-col names, such as CHOP, COP, CLOP and MOPP are common. Most include Prednisone, thus the final "P."

When remission is achieved, this does *not* mean that chemotherapy ends. In most cases, the cancer will return quickly if treatment is stopped before the end of the protocol. Just as it's known that a full course of antibiotics should be taken even if the patient is feeling better, an entire chemotherapy protocol should be completed, even if remission has been achieved.

The duration of a protocol is determined by studies conducted to find the point of diminishing returns. This is the point beyond which the average survival of dogs tested does not increase if chemotherapy treatments continue.

If a dog comes out of remission, or "relapses," an attempt is made to acquire a second remission. This time around, it's called "second line" or "rescue" chemotherapy.

If the dog comes out of remission after the protocol is completed, the same protocol may be used again. If, however, remission is achieved and the dog relapses before completing the chemotherapy protocol, the can-cer has become resistant to the drugs used to obtain the first remission and they are not used again—they have already failed. A new drug or combination of drugs is used.

In canine lymphoma, about 80 percent of the dogs achieve a first remission and about 40 percent achieve a second one. In general, the second one lasts about half as long as the first and each subsequent remission lasts a shorter period of time. Some dogs have been in and out of remission five times or more.

"Chemotherapy is not an exact science." Dr. Porzio said this many times during Bullet's treatment. If your dog reacts badly to one of the agents in your protocol, you and your oncologist can agree to customize the protocol for your dog. You can decide to give him a smaller dose of the offending agent when it appears in the schedule (a 25% discount is common). Or, you may decide to skip it entirely and replace it with a different agent.

Any deviation from a protocol should be decided on only under the expert consultation of your dog's medical team, most importantly his veterinary oncologist.

simply weaken the cells so that the next chemo agent given can kill them more effectively.

No one of these agents reliably "cures" cancer. Even though there *is* no "Magic Bullet" (except the one who used to snooze in my living room), each chemotherapy agent is effective to some degree, alone or in combination with other agents. Much of the research done involves studying the agents in different combinations and permutations to determine which grouping, in what dosages and on what time schedule has the best results. These various treatment plans are called "protocols" (see "About Protocols," page 57).

The development of a new protocol often begins at a veterinary school where veterinary oncologists select a new combination of agents, a new treatment schedule and/or a variation of dosages. Before being accepted as a viable treatment, a new protocol is evaluated in clinical trials. Clinical trials for pets with cancer are conducted at many veterinary colleges and oncology specialty practices (see "Clinical Trials," page 48).

## CHEMOTHERAPY AGENTS

Bullet's chemotherapy protocol, VELCAP-L (the "L" stands for long), had an excellent success rate but was very long and costly. Gerald S. Post, DVM,

diplomate ACVIM (oncology), examined Bullet after his chemo protocol was completed and said that the VELCAP-L protocol had fallen out of favor since Bullet's treatment, due to its cardiotoxicity (damaging to the heart).

Bullet's protocol was 75 weeks long—this is unheard of in current day protocols for dogs, most of which are 16 or 25 weeks long. This is less traumatic for the dog and less traumatic for the caretaker's finances, and Dr. Cotter explains the medical reason that chemotherapy protocols for dogs have been designed to run a shorter course:

*Most dogs—particularly those with B-cell lymphoma as opposed to T-cell—don't require 18 months of chemotherapy. We now routinely test the biopsy specimen at the time of the original diagnosis to determine which type of lymphoma is present.*

Doxorubicin (Adriamycin) is a powerful drug that is included in most chemotherapy protocols for lymphoma, hemangiosarcoma, osteosarcoma and others. This agent is cardiotoxic and eventually causes congestive heart failure. There is a lifetime maximum amount of doxorubicin that can be given, according to a dog's body surface area. Most doctors test the heart with x-ray or ultrasound before every treatment with this agent.

Some dogs tolerate doxorubicin with no ill effects and others become quite ill. If signs of early heart disease are detected, even if the lifetime maximum amount has not been given, this drug will not ever again be used on that dog.

Most protocols include Prednisone, given every day at first and then every other day. Because Prednisone can be very hard on the stomach, Alice Villalobos, DVM, director of the Animal Oncology Consultation Service in Woodland Hills and Torrance, CA, says that breaking the tablet into pieces protects the stomach lining.

Most chemotherapy agents are expelled from the dog's body through urine or feces. Some are still "active" after being expelled. Clean up vigorously, so that other dogs, cats or people do not make contact with the still-active chemical (see page 70). Wear latex gloves—active agent can be absorbed through the skin.

Protocols are modified frequently. They are modified when a dog's white blood cell count (or neutrophil count) is low. They are modified when a dog doesn't go into remission as hoped. Oncologists often improvise. They use a modified version of a widely used protocol, creating their own signature variation on a theme. Veterinarians have access to reports on the relative success rates of the various protocols.

# A DELICATE PROCEDURE

A catheter is inserted into the dog's vein. The chemotherapy agent (drug) is delivered via the catheter to ensure that the fluid does not contact the dog's body tissue outside of the vein. The chemotherapy agent is flushed through the catheter into the vein while the dog is held still.

Some chemotherapy agents that are administered intravenously can be absorbed through the skin. Members of a veterinary team administering IV (intravenous) chemotherapy wear latex gloves to ensure that the agent does not contact their skin.

A man whose dog was in chemotherapy for lymphoma applied to The Magic Bullet Fund for assistance. The veterinarian providing treatment told me that she no longer treats patients—she now works for a pharmaceutical company. She is doing her friend a favor by giving his dog low cost chemotherapy treatments. She went on to say that the treatments took place in her van, in the parking lot where they worked! The caretaker sat in the van during treatments also, holding his dog's leg still. She said that he had become anxious during one of the treatments, saying with trepidation that his dog was going to move her leg.

This is a casual treatment of a delicate procedure. I told the applicant that The Magic Bullet

Fund could not help as long as treatment was being given in this unconventional and dangerous manner.

# CHEMO LEAKS

Chemotherapy has the potential to cause a very serious complication called "extravasation," also called a "chemo leak" or a "chemo spill." Any veterinarian treating a dog with IV chemotherapy should be absolutely required to inform clients about extravasation. It is inexcusable that most caretakers who experience this nightmare have never heard of it.

Extravasation ("outside of the vein") occurs when a drop of chemo agent escapes the vein or the tubing, and contacts body tissue. Damage may not be visible right away, or for as long as 10 days.

The leaked agent proceeds on a path of destruction that is not easily stopped. The worst cases of extravasation result from a doxorubicin (Adriamycin) leak. For weeks or months, this agent continues to destroy skin, tendon and ligament. Eventually, the bone is exposed. Often, the end result is amputation. My heart goes out to anyone who has to make the heart wrenching decision of whether or not to amputate the leg of a dog who is fighting cancer.

Most agents requiring IV administration can cause extravasation, but doxorubicin is the most likely to be uncontrollable and causes the most damage. The tissue turns black, becomes very tough, dies and drops off. An open sore left that may heal, if kept free of infection.

A Magic Bullet Fund dog called Riley was in treatment for lymphoma. After her caretaker described a sore near the chemo injection site and emailed me photos of it, I called Riley's oncologist to discuss the possibility of an extravasation. The doctor felt sure that Riley had not experienced a chemo leak, but Riley's sore progressed during the following two months, looking more and more like an extravasation, until a one inch length of her leg bone was visible. Sadly, Riley succumbed to lymphoma before we were able to address the extravasation further.

Some veterinarians sedate dogs before chemotherapy; others install a "port" under the skin of a dog who won't lie still, or whose veins are difficult to catheterize. Installation of a port is a minor surgical procedure. The port requires minimal maintenance at home and can make the chemotherapy process less traumatic. Costs generally equal the costs of multiple catheterizations.

There is an excellent article about extravasation, including prevention and an effective medical response. The article is by Alice Villalobos, DVM, written for Veterinary Practice News. Please read this article and provide your veterinarian with a printout: [www.helpyourdogfightcancer.com/extravasation.html].

# BULLET'S CHEMO EXPERIENCE

During Bullet's first chemotherapy sessions, he was decidedly not the model patient. He cried, he squirmed, he growled. Once he even nipped Rod, the fellow whose job it was to get him to stay still. But, after the first few treatments, Bullet became a favorite patient. In fact, Dr. Porzio often emerged from a treatment saying that Bullet had been "an angel." He stayed still, quiet and comfortable, and give kisses to staff members holding him still. Dogs tend to become less afraid of and more agreeable to treatment in a short time.

At Bullet's first treatment, Dr. Porzio came out to tell me that he was having difficulty finding a vein in which to insert a catheter, through which the chemotherapy agent would be delivered. When I returned after 40 minutes, Bullet emerged with a shaved square on each of his four limbs.

For the following year, I asked Dr. Porzio to continue to use the vein in Bullet's left rear left leg, reshaving the same patch when necessary and allowing the fur to grow in over the other patches. I anticipated that, at some point, Dr. Porzio would tell me that the vein was no longer usable, and then we would switch to another leg.

After the first year of treatment, I asked Dr. Porzio to switch to the right rear leg and give the left rear vein a rest. Eventually, a vein used repeatedly may collapse or become irritated and I feared that we were pushing our luck.

Any veterinarian who treated Bullet knew I was strongly against his fur being shaved unnecessarily. It's important to preserve the beauty and natural integrity of the animal whenever possible.

An ultrasound examination of Bullet's heart was performed before each treatment with doxorubicin. Although no signs of early heart disease were detected, Bullet consistently became very ill from this agent. I chose to discontinue the inclusion of Adriamycin in Bullet's protocol long before his lifetime maximum quantity was reached. When it came up in the protocol, another agent was substituted.

Some veterinarians prefer to treat a fasted dog. If your oncologist has no objections, encourage your dog to drink water before IV chemotherapy treatments. This will dilate his veins and make the insertion of the catheter simpler for the doctor and less traumatic for your dog.

*Notes*

# SIDE EFFECTS

6

*Buckle up and hold on tight!*
*The canine cancer journey can be a roller coaster ride.*
*On bad days, believe that tomorrow will be bright*
*And relish the good days like there's no tomorrow.*

Every prescription drug has a set of related side effects. Some are common and others occurred only in a small percentage of the test population. Likewise, each chemotherapy agent has a set of reactions that were experienced by a certain percentage of clinical trial participants.

Still, these are only statistics. Some dogs are overly sensitive to all of the agents and become ill from each treatment. Others suffer side effects only to particular agents. Still others seem immune to all side effects from any agent and withstand every treatment without any sign of illness.

Your dog may not have typical reactions to chemotherapy treatments. He may have reactions not included in the list of common side effects.

When serious side effects do occur, dosages are decreased in subsequent treatments and, more often than not, the dog tolerates the lower dose. Most dogs will react more or less consistently to each chemotherapy agent. After your dog's first treatment with each agent, you'll be prepared for his reaction the next time this agent is given.

If your dog has an adverse reaction to a chemotherapy treatment, don't hesitate to inform your veterinarian or oncologist right away. He might be able to provide medication, or there might be something you can do at home to stop the reaction. He might say to bring your pet into the clinic right away or not to worry because the reaction is normal and is not dangerous.

# KEEP YOUR DOG HEALTHY DURING CHEMOTHERAPY

*by Dr. Kevin A. Hahn*

Your dog has cancer and you feel helpless. His body is turning against itself and your veterinary oncologist has said that nothing can be done to cure your dog but chemotherapy may delay the inevitable.

Are you helpless? No! There are measures that you and your veterinary team can take to minimize chemotherapy side effects and allow your dog to enjoy a longer, better quality life.

Chemotherapy side effects occur because the agents are designed to kill rapidly growing cells. The vast majority of cells killed are cancer cells. However, bone marrow and cells of the intestinal lining also grow rapidly and are killed by chemotherapy as innocent bystanders.

Bone marrow and the intestine produce a certain percentage of new cells every day and those cells are "reserved" to be used by the body 1 to 3 days later. For this reason, most complications from chemotherapy occur 1 to 3 days after treatment.

▸ **Be Observant.** Be sure to report all chemotherapy side effects to your veterinarian. If treatment is needed, it should begin as early as possible in order to get the best result.

▸ **Check for Fever.** If your dog seems tired, lethargic or weak, don't rely on body warmth, a wet or dry nose or panting—take his rectal temperature. Fever may be caused by low white blood cell count (neutropenia) or by the death of tumor cells (non-infectious inflammation) and may be treated with intravenous fluids or antibiotics. Normal temperature in a dog ranges from 100.0 to 103.5 degrees Fahrenheit.

▸ **Feed Wisely.** There's no universally accepted "good diet" for pets on chemotherapy. A well-balanced diet that is easy to digest (requiring less work from the intestine), easily absorbed (generating less stool, hence less diarrhea) and high in calories (to avoid weight loss and protein loss) is best.

The recommended diet is low in carbohydrates, high in the non-inflammatory fats (Omega 3 fatty acids or fish oils) and provides good quality protein (from egg or poultry products). Consult with your veterinary team about the commercial, prescription or homemade diet that's right for your pet's body condition, breed and diagnosis.

Alternative treatments and immune stimulants may be helpful, but always consult with your veterinarian and provide a list of all supplements at each visit. Some may worsen side effects of chemotherapy or interfere with treatment.

▸ **Promote Wellness.** Some serious complications can arise long after the completion of chemotherapy. Because these delayed problems may occur months to years after treatment and because they often go unnoticed, regular veterinary examinations are warranted. Other health-care measures, including heartworm prevention and flea control, are still necessary.

The essential rule for good home care is "when in doubt, check it out." Tell your veterinary team about every concern that you have.

*Kevin A. Hahn, DVM, PhD, diplomate ACVIM (Oncology), PhD, practicing in Houston and San Antonio, Texas.*

Now that you have a whole "team" of experts contributing to your dog's well-being, you'll learn which team member or members to call on for assistance when a problem arises. Call one or all—in time, you'll learn who is most accessible and who has the best solutions. Don't forget to make a notation in your log with all of the details of the episode, including what it was that finally helped.

The following section is an overview of common side effects, each followed by some of the available remedies. This is not by any means a comprehensive list. You can find more information about supplements at the end of the book in "Resources" on page 130, and don't forget to use the special offer coupons in the color plate.

### VOMITING AND NAUSEA

▸ Watch for signs of dehydration. To test, pick up the skin on the scruff of your dog's neck, where a pup's mother (that is, his genetic mother) would grab on to carry the pup. Then let go. If the skin doesn't fall down flat on your dog's neck within a few seconds, he may be dehydrated and you should call your veterinarian. Call your veterinarian if there is any blood in the vomitus, if vomiting persists for more than two days or if your dog vomits more than three times in a 24-hour period.

▸ The vomitus may contain toxic chemicals that were not absorbed into your dog's system. Clean up as best you can wearing protective gloves. Then, dissipate the vomitus by pouring water over it so that other animals don't eat it.

▸ Dr. Cotter says that antiemetics can prevent vomiting in dogs undergoing chemotherapy. If your dog vomits after a treatment, report this to your oncologist. Before the next treatment that includes the offending agent, he can pre-treat your dog with antiemetics.

*Prescription (Rx): Your veterinarian may prescribe an antinausea (antiemetic) drug such as Cerenia™, Reglan®. Zofran® or Anzemet®.*

*Over The Counter (OTC): PeptoBismol® (check with your veterinarian first), particularly after chemotherapy agent doxorubicin is given.*

*Pepcid AC® (check with your veterinarian first)*

*Other: Ginger is well known as a natural remedy for nausea*

*Pumpkin may help when your pup is nauseous. Canned mashed pumpkin can easily be found in any supermarket.*

*L-Glutamine: If your dog takes this regularly, you can double the amount while vomiting persists. (Do not give your dog L-Glutamine if he has epilepsy or is taking anti-seizure medication.)*

*Nux Vomica 6C*

### DIARRHEA

▸ Again, clean up!

▸ Watch for mucous (a loose stool that glistens and/or hangs before falling to the ground; a liquid stool that's shiny with consistency of uncooked egg white). If you suspect there is mucous in your dog's stools, report this to your veterinarian.

▸ Projectile diarrhea: This is a shocking occurrence for the caretaker and, I can only surmise, for the dog. Try to stay out of the spray zone—otherwise, treat the same as ordinary diarrhea.

*Rx: Metronidazole (Flagyl®) to decrease inflammation.*

*OTC: PeptoBismol; Imodium®; Lomotil. Check with your veterinarian before giving these remedies.*

*Other: Do not give vitamin C or CoQ10.*

*Temporarily decrease oil (fatty acids) in food.*

*L-Glutamine: \*Do not give L-Glutamine if your dog has epilepsy or is taking antiseizure medication.*

*Acidophilus and bifidus: As chewable tablets or in organic yogurt.*

*Potato, brown rice, sweet potato, pumpkin: Only until the diarrhea stops.*

*Pectin: Mix a teaspoon of powdered pectin with filtered water in a needle-less syringe and empty it slowly into your dog's mouth.*

*High-fiber bran cereal: Sprinkled it onto a meal or mix with water as above.*

### BLOODY DIARRHEA

▸ The lining of a dog's intestines can be damaged by chemotherapy agents. If you see blood in your dog's stool, notify your veterinary oncologist immediately and make a note in your log. If bleeding occurs in the intestines, the stool may appear black rather than red because of the distance between the source and the exit point.

If the bleeding doesn't stop within two days (or sooner if severe), an examination will be necessary.

*Remedies: Same as those listed for diarrhea.*

### NOT EATING

▸ Loss of appetite can indicate the presence of infection. Check your dog's temperature and alert your veterinarian if it is above 103 degrees Fahrenheit.

▸ Don't panic, but do try anything and everything. Start with foods that are healthy and cancer-conscious, but resort to anything. The longer he doesn't eat, the less inclined he will be to start eating—in other words, "not eating" can become habitual.

▸ Feed Frozen. Heating food to combat nausea is often recommended but in my experience has not been effective. I've had great success with frozen or semi-frozen food (see "Feeding Frozen," page 80).

*Rx: Antiemetics may be prescribed since loss of appetite may be due to nausea.*

*OTC: Pepcid AC, Rescue Remedy*

*Other: Frozen fish, cottage cheese, ginger, garlic*

### "FLAT OUT"

When a dog is nonresponsive, not eating and hardly moving, I call this condition "flat out." Dr. Ruslander advises that this condition is important because,

> *This could represent neutropenia [low neutrophil count—neutrophils are a type of WBC] or sepsis [high levels of toxin in the blood], which is the most concerning acute side effect that veterinary oncologists worry about. If the dog is febrile (has a temperature above 103 degrees F.), this is a life-threatening emergency.*

Dr. Cotter says that when a dog is febrile, bactericidal antibiotics such as a combination of gentamicin and cephalothin or fluoroquinolones are given intravenously until the neutrophil count rises. In most cases, this occurs within 2 to 3 days.

*Your veterinarian will check your dog's white blood cell count and neutrophil count.*

*Check your dog's temperature.*

*Get him to eat! Try anything and everything. Appetite enhancers are generally not effective in dogs.*

*Rescue Remedy, Vitamin B-12*

### DIFFICULTY BREATHING

Some dogs have allergic reactions to certain chemotherapy agents in the form of respiratory distress. This may manifest as rasping, wheezing or reverse sneezing. Notify your oncologist or your veterinarian right away—anaphylactic shock is possible and can be fatal. If the cause is a sensitivity to a particular chemotherapy agent, the dosage of the agent may be decreased. If the symptoms are caused by an allergic reaction, use of the agent is discontinued entirely.

*Inform your veterinarian immediately*

*Rx: Clavamox, one of the newer "designer" antibiotics, controlled this reaction very effectively for Bullet. Dr. Cotter says that antibiotics will help resolve this condition if it's caused by a respiratory infection such as pneumonia.*

### SWELLING

This may signal an allergic reaction to a chemotherapy agent or to the long-term use of Prednisone. Swelling may also be caused by edema due to a tumor or by heart failure.

*Inform your veterinarian immediately*

### LOW WHITE BLOOD CELL COUNT

A CBC (Complete Blood Count) will be done regularly while your dog is in chemotherapy. Cut-off points vary but a white blood cell count lower than about 3,000 and/or neutrophil count lower than about 2,000 may prompt your oncologist to suspend chemotherapy temporarily.

*Rx: Antibiotics*

*Neupogen® (Filgrastim) may be prescribed to increase the number of neutrophils in the blood.*

*Other: Cancer-dog caretakers have reported that adding rinsed light red kidney beans to their dog's food between chemotherapy treatments helps to keep the white blood cell count from dropping.*

### ANEMIA

Although anemia (insufficient red blood cell count) is not a typical chemotherapy side effect, many dogs in cancer treatment become mildly anemic as a reaction to the immunosuppressive nature of chemotherapy. However, if the cancer has infiltrated the bone marrow and is not in remission, the red cells, white cells and platelets all become insufficient. The prognosis in this situation is very poor.

*Rx: Procrit® is often prescribed*

*Aranesp® (darbepoetin alfa) treats anemia caused by chemotherapy*

### NEUROPATHY

Chemotherapy agents and radiation therapy can both cause neuropathy in a limb, where nerve coatings are stripped away from the nerves. This causes numbness and/or pain and usually (but not always) resolves after the cause is removed. Watch your dog for signs such as limping, knuckling or inability to walk. Agents that can cause neuropathy include carboplatin, vincristine, cisplatin and paclitaxel.

*L-Glutamine*

### HAIR LOSS

Fur clipped or shaved during chemotherapy will grow back, but more slowly than normal. When shaving is unavoidable, ask team members not to shave any more of your dog's coat than is absolutely necessary. Bullet's team members were aware of my opposition to unnecessary shaving or clipping and went out of their way to oblige me. If your dog's coat is like Samson's long locks, appeal to your dog's doctors to shave sparingly.

Dogs don't typically lose their hair during chemotherapy as do humans (with few exceptions, including poodles, other dogs that have "hair" rather than "fur" and some terriers). This is because hair growth for most dogs is seasonal, not continual. It is common, however, for dogs to lose their whiskers early on and to experience some hair loss if the chemotherapy continues for more than a few months.

*Brush well to remove loose hair/fur*

*Nettles (dry herb flakes, crumbled on food)*

*Silica 500 supplement (health food store)*

# DON'T PANIC!

If your dog doesn't tolerate chemotherapy, you and your veterinary oncologist will probably agree to postpone treatment until your dog has recovered from side effects. Treat the symptoms, make your dog as comfortable as possible and hope for a turnaround. Make use of your team members and pay attention to your own instincts, based on your intimate knowledge of your dog.

### DECISION OPTIONS WITH SEVERE SIDE EFFECTS

▸ Continue treatment according to protocol in hopes that your dog will better tolerate subsequent treatments.

▸ Continue treatment with revisions to the protocol, including amounts and types of agents used and/or the scheduling of treatments. If there is one specific chemotherapy agent that causes severe side effects in your dog, that agent can be omitted from the protocol and replaced with another or the dosage of the agent can be reduced in future treatments.

▸ Stop current treatment. Initiate a different treatment, such as a standard but less widely used treatment for the condition, an alternative therapy or a therapy in clinical trials.

▸ Stop treatment and provide palliative care.

If your dog doesn't respond to treatment as hoped and remission is not achieved, your veterinary oncologist may employ other agents or perhaps, depending on the type and location of the cancer, other therapies in an attempt to induce remission. Ultimately, if this fails, he will probably provide you with a new prognosis and a recommendation for palliative care.

At this point, you might make the decision to stop fighting and focus instead on maximizing your dog's quality of life. Remember that many dogs outlive their prognoses.

But, if you're not ready to give up the fight, there are still a few options that you can explore. Clinical trials, for example, often seek out dogs that have been resistant to standard therapies. Your holistic veterinarian can provide a selection of alternative therapies to choose from. You can also explore the library and the Internet for new approaches.

# CHEMOTHERAPY AGENTS AND SIDE EFFECTS [1]

| GENERIC NAME (BRAND NAME) | CANCER TYPE | HOW GIVEN | CLEARED VIA WITHIN (APPROX) | COMMON SIDE EFFECTS |
|---|---|---|---|---|
| actinomycin-D (Cosmegen) | LSA | IV | Urine, feces [7 days] | Vessels, myelosuppression, G.I., Extravasation |
| asparaginase (Elspar®) (L-asparaginase) | LSA, Leukemia | SubQ | [1 day*] | Anaphylaxis, mild myelosuppression * Pretreat: Benadryl® |
| bleomycin (Blenoxane®) | Carcinomas, LSA, Leukemia | SubQ | Urine [3 hrs*] Active | Mild myelosuppression, Kidney, Liver |
| busulfan (Busulfex®) | Myeloblastic Leukemia | Oral | Urine [2.5 hours] | Myelosuppression, lower G.I. |
| capecytabine (Xeloda®) | Carcinoma, Mammary, HSA | Oral | Urine [1 day] | Myelosuppression, G.I., Neurological |
| carboplatin (Paraplatin®) | Osteosarcoma, Melanoma | IV infusion | Urine [1 day*] Active | Myelosuppression, G.I., Allergy |
| chlorambucil (Leukeran®) | LSA, Leukemia, STT, MCT | Oral | Urine [1 day*] | Moderate myelosuppression; G.I. |
| cisplatin (Platinol®) | Osteosarcoma, Melanoma | IV infusion | Urine [3 days] Active | Kidney Failure; Severe myelosuppression, G.I. *Pretreat: IV fluid diuresis; Zofran® |
| cyclophosphamide (Cytoxan®) | LSA, Leukemia, STT | Oral; IV | Urine [3 days] | Severe myelosuppression, G.I., Bleeding Cystitis * With treatment: oral fluids, Prednisone |
| cytosine (Cytosar-U®) | Leukemia | SubQ | Urine [1 day*] | Severe myelosuppression, G.I. |
| dacarbazine (DTIC-Dome®) | Relapsed LSA | IV | Urine | Severe Vomiting, Myelosuppression |
| doxorubicin (Adriamycin®) epirubicin idarubicin (Idamycin PFS) | LSA, STT, many types of cancer " Leukemia | IV infusion IV infusion IV / Oral | Feces [7 days] Active | Severe myelosuppression, G.I., Anaphylaxis, Cardiomyopathy, Extravasation * Pretreat: Benadryl, Cerenia |
| 5-FU (5-Fluorouracil®) | STT | IV / Intralesional | Urine [20 minutes] | Seizures, Neurological, Moderate myelosuppression |
| gemcitabine HCl (Gemzar®) | Pancreatic/Hepatocellular Carcinomas | IV | Urine [3-4 days] | Myelosuppression, Vomiting, Anaphylaxis |
| hydroxyurea (Hydrea®) | Leukemia | Oral | Urine [Peak 1-4 hrs*] | Severe myelosuppression |
| ifosfamide (Ifex®) | many | IV infusion | Urnie [7 days] | Myelosuppression; Neurological |
| interferon (Intron-A®; Roferon-A®) | Leukemia, Melanoma, others | IV | Urine [1 day] | Liver * Pretreat: Benadryl |
| lomustine (CEENU®) (CCNU) | Relapsed LSA, MCT | Oral / IV | Urine [1 day*] | Myelosuppression, G.I., Lungs. Liver |

| | | | | |
|---|---|---|---|---|
| melphalan (Alkeran®) | Leukemia | Oral; IV | Urine [7 days*] | Moderate myelosuppression |
| methotrexate (Trexall®) | LSA, Leukemia | IV | Urine [1 day*] | Moderate myelosuppression, G.I. |
| mitoxantrone (Novantrone®) | LSA, STT | IV infusion | Urine [5 days] Feces [7 days] | Myelosuppression, Anaphylaxis, G.I. |
| mustargen (Mechlorethamine®) | LSA. Leukemia | IV | Urine [immediate] | Extravasation, Severe Myelosuppression, G.I. |
| pacitaxel (Taxol®) | Osteosarcoma and others | IV infusion | Feces [5 days] | Anemia, G.I., Neurological *Pretreat: Benadryl, Cerenia |
| piroxicam (Feldene®) | TCC, CMM, Carciomas, HSA | Oral | Urine, Feces [50 hrs*] | G.I. Ulceration; Anemia, Platelets |
| Prednisone; prednisolone | LSA, Leukemia, Insulinoma | Oral | [4 hours] | Thirst & Urination, Panting, weakness, Cushings. Mild myelosuppression |
| tamoxifen (Nolvadex®) | Mammary, Brain & MDR Tumors | Oral | Feces [5-7 days*] | Vaginal discharge, Pyometra in females |
| vinblastine (Velban®) | LSA, Leukemia, MCT, STT | IV infusion | Feces [3 days*] | Severe myelosuppression, G.I. |
| vincristine (Oncovin®) | LSA, Leukemia, MCT, STT | IV | Urine [4 days] Feces [7 days] | Mild-moderate myelosuppression, G.I., Neurological, Extravasation |

Cancer Type: **LSA**=Lymphoma; **CMM**=Canine Malignant Melanoma; **TCC**=Transitional Cell Carcinoma; **STT**=Soft Tissue Tumors. **MCT**=Mast Cell Tumor; HSA=Henangiosarcoma

How Given: **SubQ**=subcutaneous injection; **IV**=intravenous; **IM**=Intramuscular injection.

* Asterisked clearance times apply to human metabolization (I was unable to find canine-specific times). May be shorter or equal in the canine.

Side Effects: **Myelosuppression**=Bone marrow unable to create new blood cells; **G.I.**=Gastrointestinal; **Anaphylaxis**=Severe allergic reaction

## CHEMO NOTES

▸ Every dog reacts differently to each chemo drug. Don't anticipate a crash just because of a drug's "reputation." Don't be caught off guard if your dog has effects form a "friendly" agent.

▸ Ask your doctor to pretreat with Benadryl and/or anti-emetics to help avoid side effects.

▸ Most treatments take 20 minutes to 2 hours.

▸ Watch for extravasations! Examine injection sites closely and report sores or eruptions to the doctor immediately.

▸ Protocols can be altered. Dosages are reduced and schedules extended as needed.

▸ Treatments halted/postponed: The most common cause is low white blood cell count (WBC) and neutrophils (polys, absolute polys or ANC [absolute neutrophil count]).

▸ Don't panic if treatment is halted! This is very common. WBC usually recovers in 1-2 weeks.

▸ Watch for neuropathy. If your dog is limping or knuckling, or reluctant to be active, tell your doctor.

▸ If your dog cannot tolerate chemo, be prepared to switch to palliative care.

Not Today and Not Without a Fight!

# BULLET'S SIDE EFFECTS

For Bullet, chemotherapy began with a treatment of doxorubicin. He showed no reaction at all except that he threw up lots of clear fluid once, a day later. I remember vividly because I was in the middle of a phone consult with Tina Aiken, a holistic veterinarian at Dr. Marty Goldstein's office who has been immensely helpful throughout. Bullet had a second doxorubicin treatment a week later and this time he became extremely ill. Bullet didn't eat for nearly two weeks. He was basically flat out 24/7, sometimes crying quietly. He needed my help to go outside to pee. There was blood in his stool and he was vomiting. I wondered if I was being unkind by keeping him alive.

Once, upon seeing Bullet's condition, a friend said, "You know, many people whose pets have cancer feel that euthanasia's a kinder option than treatment." Her message was clear and indeed I did question my decision to keep going then (and many other times when Bullet became ill), but in each case I decided "not yet." I had no way of knowing that Bullet would survive the episode. If he had not, would my decision have been the wrong one? Perhaps in retrospect it would have been, but in the absence of a crystal ball, I simply had to trust my instincts.

Bullet and I weathered a number of seemingly hopeless setbacks. With each new setback, I knew that this time could turn out to be the one that Bullet would not survive. But I stored that understanding in the back of my mind and continued to believe, each time, that he would recover and simply went about taking care of him the best I could.

As for side effects, Bullet never once came out of the clinic after a chemotherapy treatment ill. I waited for him because my schedule allowed it and because I wanted to avoid making him wait in a cage, since he was cage-protective. At the end of every treatment, Bullet came trotting out happily. When he suffered side effects, the symptoms appeared 5 to 10 days after a treatment.

The first time Bullet had what I call a "flat out" reaction, he was practically motionless, lying on his side for nearly two weeks. He would get up only if I first lifted him to a half-standing position and he would not eat. He looked deflated. I thought that it would be a miracle if he pulled through.

Whenever Bullet had a flat out day during his protocol, Dr. Porzio or Dr. Hoskins would first ensure that he did not have a fever, that his white blood cell count (WBC) was adequate and that he was not dehydrated. After that, I simply waited it out and did what I could to help him recover.

I tried feeding him anything and everything, but he had no interest whatsoever in food. Bullet lost 15 pounds during those two weeks, dropping from 85 pounds to 70. I have no doubt that the discovery of Bully's Frozen Food Diet saved his life (see "Feeding Frozen," page 82).

I discovered one other method to get Bullet to eat—I don't have a clue how I came across it. I placed the food bowl within Bullet's reach and I inserted a finger into his ear (sometimes one in each ear) and rubbed gently, back and forth. Where? Somewhere within the nooks and crannies. I found a particular pot that seemed to prompt a reflexive eating response! No guarantees, but perhaps it will work for your dog, too.

After Bullet's first dramatic weight loss, I made a decision to KEEP HIM FAT, and this remained a mantra throughout. I tried to maintain him at about five pounds over what I considered to be his perfect weight. My thinking was that I would not panic about a one- or two-day fast if he had a few extra pounds on him.

Vomiting wasn't a problem for Bullet. He vomited once after about a third of the chemotherapy treatments and two or three times after a few treatments. The vomitus usually consisted of a large volume of clear fluid, which I cleaned up as best I could.

Bullet lost all of his whiskers at month #3 of his chemotherapy protocol, but the rest of his coat remained intact until month 17. At that time, with only one month of chemotherapy left, his entire undercoat fell out suddenly, in handfuls. For the first time in his life, Bullet was showing pink skin on his belly.

I added supplements thought to promote hair growth to his regimen and the undercoat grew back nicely. Then, just as his undercoat was growing in again, his guardhair coat dropped out. Bullet's head and neck retained the double coat typical of a Northern breed dog, but the rest of his body was furred only with a soft, downy undercoat. The next time we went to Dr. Porzio's office for a chemotherapy treatment, the doctor saw Bullet and exclaimed, "Hey, the Bullet looks like a giant chinchilla!"

For the rest of his life, Bullet had no guardhair coat except around his neck. His body was soft as cotton and I added the nickname, "Bunny Boy" to the list of endearments. I missed watching my fingers disappear into his deep, luxurious fur but, all in all, this was a very small price to pay for four and a half years on borrowed time!

*Notes*

# WHAT'S FOR DINNER?

*A healthy diet is important for any dog.*
*For a dog with cancer, a well researched diet*
*that feeds the patient and not the cancer is essential.*

Extensive research has been done toward understanding the relationship between nutrition and canine cancer. The consensus is that dietary intake is a significant factor in the survival of the cancer patient.

A great deal of what's known about the effect of diet on canine cancer is known due to research by Gregory K. Ogilvie, DVM, diplomate ACVIM (Internal Medicine and Oncology), at Colorado State University College of Veterinary Medicine and Biomedical Sciences. Dr. Ogilvie's team and a team from Hill's Pet Nutrition, Inc.®, worked together to develop Prescription Diet® Canine n/d®, currently the only commercial food formulated specifically for dogs with cancer[1].

The n/d diet was formulated according to Dr. Ogilvie's findings. Studies show that dogs with lymphoma in chemotherapy and dogs with nasal or oral cancer in radiation therapy who eat n/d have a significantly longer survival rate than those who eat other commercially produced dog foods. Very possibly, dogs with any type of cancer would benefit from n/d—other cancers have simply not been tested.

Some caretakers feed cancer dogs Innova Evo® by Natura Pet Products®, an excellent natural food for dogs but with a carbohydrate content of 12 percent (from fruits and potatoes).[2] For dogs who are fed foods other than n/d, L-Arginine can be added in supplement form.

Current dietary guidelines for dogs with cancer are based on two of Dr. Ogilvie's findings. In broad strokes: 1) Cancer cells readily metabolize carbohydrates and 2) Cancer cells are unable to metabolize fats. Because the goal is to feed the patient and not the cancer, we provide those nutrients that the patient is able to utilize and that cancer cells are unable to utilize (i.e., certain fatty acids) and withhold those that the cancer cells can utilize, thereby depriving the patient of those nutrients (i.e., carbohydrates). It seems certain that a diet high in Omega 3 fatty acids and low in carbohydrates will improve a dog's prognosis and his chance of achieving remission or cure.

A high-fat diet contains Omega 3 fatty acids. Flax seed oil, cod liver oil and fish oil are at the top of this list. Flax seed oil has the highest O-3 fatty acid content, but its Omega 6 fatty acids content is fairly high. When O-3 fatty acids are used nutritionally or in supplement form, antioxidants such as vitamin E should be given as well.[3]

A diet low in carbohydrates omits foods that contain sugar or starch such as fruits, some vegetables, most grains, potatoes and legumes. Dog biscuits are often high in carbohydrates, so if you feel that they are essential in maintaining your dog's quality of life, then choose a biscuit with a low carbohydrate content.

*Cancer Cachexia* (ka-KEX-ia) is a condition that can develop secondary to cancer. A cachectic dog experiences drastic and progressive weight loss regardless of the quality or quantity of food eaten. He becomes unable to metabolize nutrients and, eventually, reaches a state of severe malnutrition. Once cachexia has developed, it is extremely hard to reverse. Often a dog will have a cure or remission from cancer and die from cachexia. Studies indicate that a low carbohydrate, high fat diet may, in some way, protect a dog from cachexia and decrease the likelihood of a dog with cancer developing cancer cachexia.[4]

*Cancer anorexia* can also develop secondary to cancer. It's similar to cachexia in that the dog undergoes extreme weight loss, but in this case the weight loss is due to the dog's refusal to eat. Cancer anorexia can be reversed more easily than cancer cachexia.

# FEEDING NATURALLY

Dogs have been domesticated for over 14,000 years but the dog food industry has been around less than a century. Technology stepped in to save caretakers time—to make feeding as simple, tidy and effortless as pouring pellets into a bowl. It's easier for us, but is it healthy for our pets?

# Bullet's Cancer Diet

## A Sampling of Ingredients

...and an illustrated food preparation
plan to get you started, pages C2-C4.

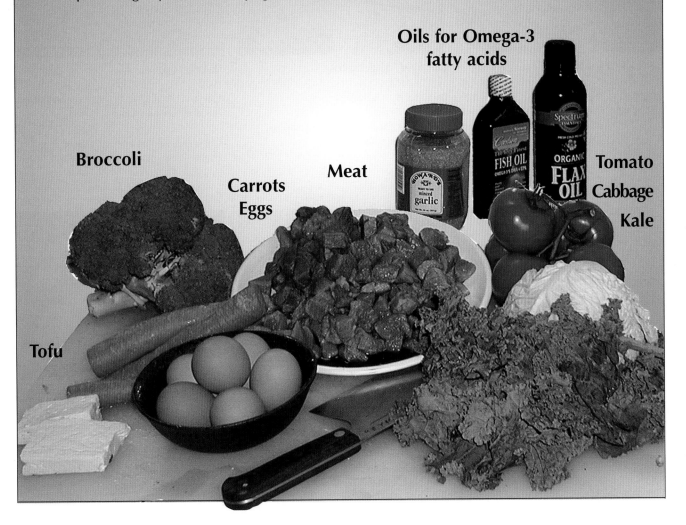

Oils for Omega-3 fatty acids

Broccoli

Carrots

Eggs

Meat

Tomato

Cabbage

Kale

Tofu

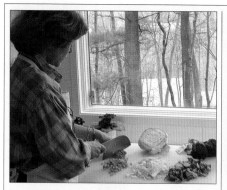

### 1. "Dry" Vegetables
Use broccoli and a cabbage-family vegetable. Kale, celery, carrots and other vegetables can be used as well.

**Steam or food-process vegetables.
Set aside.**

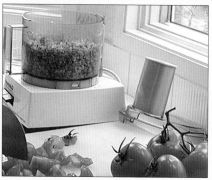

### 2. "Wet" Vegetables
Tomatoes contain antioxidants, and are high in Vitamin C.

**Steam or food-process vegetables.
Add to vegetable bowl.**

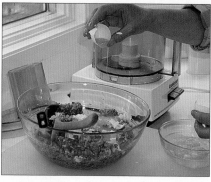

### 3. Egg Yolks
Add yolks into the vegetable bowl. Drop whites and crumbled shells into another bowl to be cooked.

**Cook egg whites and crumbled egg shells—they may deplete biotin.**

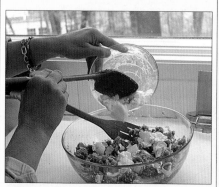

### 4. Egg Whites and Shells
Cook the whites and crumbled shells until the egg-white is solid enough to cut with a fork.

**Add to vegetable bowl.**

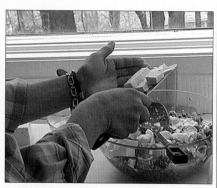

### 5. Tofu
Tofu is a very good source of protein. It may be added into the combination at any point of the process.

**After adding all ingredients except meat and oils, hand mix as though tossing a salad.**

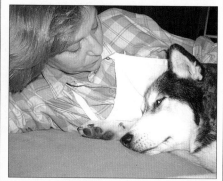

### 6. Take a Break!
If your dog works as hard as Bullet did, he's likely exhausted by now.

**You can divide your work into two parts by stopping at this point—just cover and refrigerate the bowl overnight.**

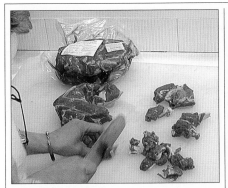

### 7. Prepare Meat
Cube the meat into bite-sized pieces. Use beef, chicken, turkey or fish. Meat may be cooked or raw.

**Put cubed meat into a bowl and retrieve the vegetable bowl from the refrigerator.**

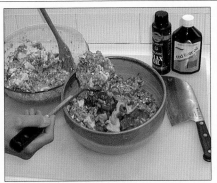

### 8. Combine Vegetables and Meat
Add processed or cooked vegetables to the meat so that about ¼ of the contents is vegetable and ¾ is meat.

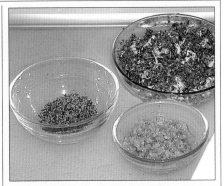

### 9. Add Flax Seeds and Garlic
Add flax seeds (be sure they're hulled or milled) and garlic.

**Add about 1 tsp flax seeds and about a clove of garlic per pound of meat.**

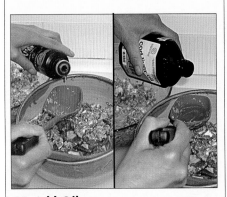

### 10. Add Oils
Use about 2 Tbs of oil per pound of meat.

**I confess, I didn't actually measure. I added oils watched to see how much the meat absorbed.**

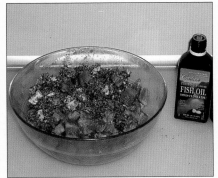

### 11. Vary Types of Oils
Flax seed, fish, salmon, cod liver and olive oil are all high in Omega N-3 fatty acids. I recommend a rotation. **I used flax seed oil most consistently throughout Bullet's cancer treatment.**

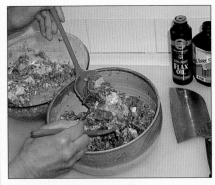

### 12. Hand Mix (toss) all
This is another good stopping point. If necessary, you can cover and refrigerate the bowls overnight.

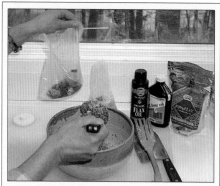

**13. Scoop into Plastic Bags**
Each storage bag should contain no more than three days worth of food.

**Keep one bag in the refrigerator. When you finish a bag, move a new one from freezer to refrigerator.**

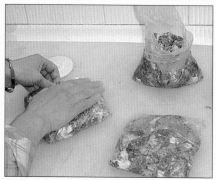

**14. Flatten Bags**
Frozen food should not be exposed to air. After filling a bag, squeeze the air out of it and pat it down flat.

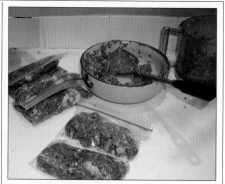

**15. Subdivide bags**
You can subdivide bags to hold one meal each.

**To subdivide, use the bags with air-tight closures—not fold-over sandwich bags.**

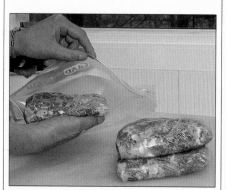

**16. Double-Bag It**
Keep bags free of air and the freezer free of drippings—pack small bags into a large one with air-tight closure.

**If you're double-bagging, sandwich bags work fine for the inner package.**

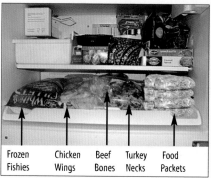

Frozen Fishies   Chicken Wings   Beef Bones   Turkey Necks   Food Packets

**17. Freeze It**
The bottom shelf of my freezer belonged to Bullet. Some dogs come running when they hear the sound of a can opener. Not my Bullet—he came running to the sound of the freezer door opening.

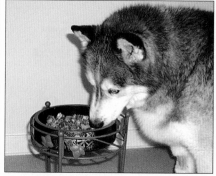

**18. Thaw and serve!**
At serving time, add n/d, yogurt, cottage cheese and/or supplements and medications.

**Add filtered or bottled water to the food if your dog isn't drinking enough water.**

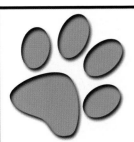
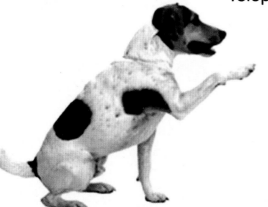

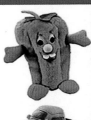

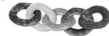
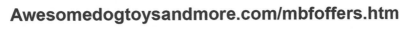
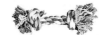

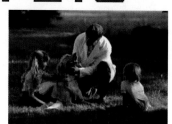
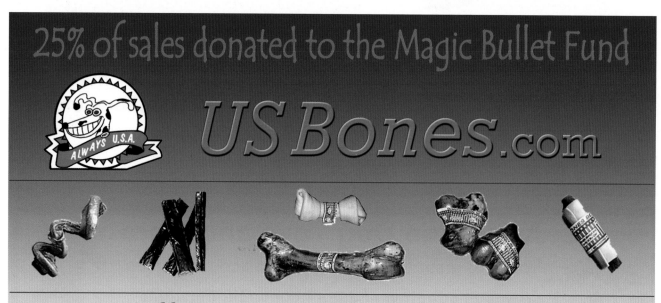

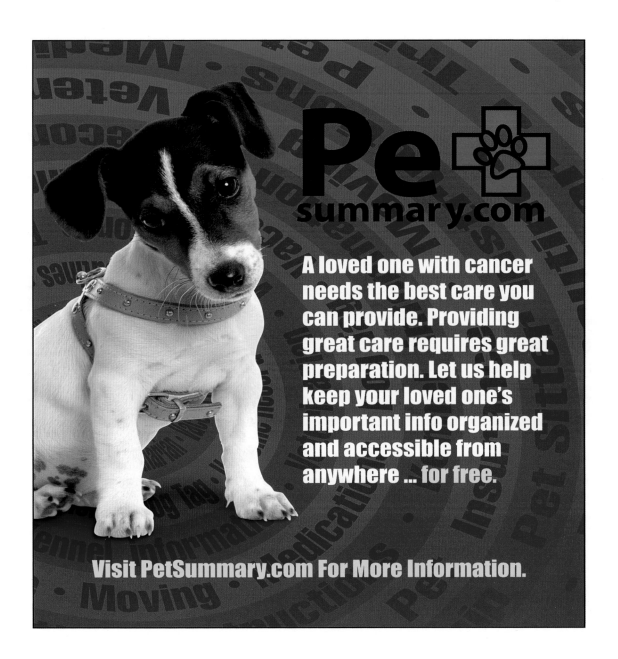

Pe<sup></sup>
summary.com

A loved one with cancer needs the best care you can provide. Providing great care requires great preparation. Let us help keep your loved one's important info organized and accessible from anywhere ... for free.

Visit PetSummary.com For More Information.

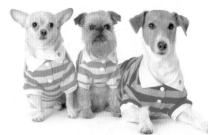
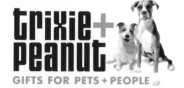
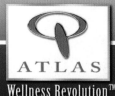

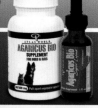
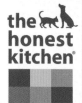
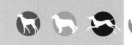
C8          *Offers included for your consideration. The author and publisher do not endorse or guarantee any products.*

Many commercially produced dog foods are comprised of poor quality ingredients that have been cooked at extremely high temperatures, thus destroying much or all natural nutritional content. Nutrients listed on the product label are in the food only because they have been added back in after processing, as additives. If you wish to feed "dog food" to your dog with cancer, find one with a low carbohydrate content. You may have to call the manufacturer to get this information.

But there is an alternative. More and more dog caretakers are choosing not to feed their pets canned or bagged food. You can feed your dog "real" food—i.e, whole foods, human grade foods, unprocessed foods.

You may be thinking of the warnings you've undoubtedly heard. *"Don't feed your pets table food—it may kill them!"* It may or may not, depending of course on what you eat! I'm not suggesting that you feed your dog a diet of table scraps or serve him up a dish of whatever you and your family are having for breakfast, lunch and dinner.

A natural or "wild-type" diet for a dog does not involve feeding your dog the food that you eat. It means providing him with a diet that mimics what a dog (or a wolf, with a nearly identical genetic makeup to the dog) eats in the wild.

The canid in the wild doesn't intentionally eat fruits and vegetables. He does, however, eat the stomach and intestines of his prey, which may contain partially digested fruits and vegetables. The wild-*type* diet mimics this by including fruits and vegetables that have been well cooked or pulverized in a food processor. This enables a dog's digestive system to extract the nutrients.

Wolf biologist L. David Mech says that the stomach of the prey is rarely eaten by the predator wolf. Nonetheless, most wild-type canine diets include pulverized or steamed vegetables.[5]

The meat in a *truly* wild diet comes from deer, caribou, mice and other animals that are natural prey of the wolf. Muscle meat and organs, some cartilage and bone are all consumed. As for food preparation, the canine hunter certainly doesn't build a fire and cook his kill—he eats it raw.

## IS A RAW DIET SAFE?

The wild canine has a digestive tract and digestive acids that enable him to process raw meat. The practice of feeding raw meat to our not-so-wild dogs has gained popularity in recent years, but is still controversial among veterinarians. In general, as might be expected, traditional veterinarians are against it and holistic veterinarians for it. Is the domestic canine susceptible to bacterium such as *salmonella* and *E. coli*? Some veterinarians say that dogs are invulnerable to these "bugs," while others disagree. Still others claim that it's a moot point so long as the food is frozen before serving.

I froze Bullet's Cancer Diet before serving it, to abolish bacteria in the raw meat. While preparing Bullet's food, however, I would sometimes sneak him tidbits of raw meat not yet frozen. In over three years, including during the entire course of chemotherapy, he never suffered any ill effects.

If you switch your dog to a raw diet, do so gradually. If any vomiting or diarrhea results, just return to a cooked or processed diet. Some dogs don't tolerate raw food and some caretakers don't feel comfortable serving it. It's a personal decision for you and your dog to make. All of the ingredients in Bullet's Cancer Diet were raw, but the diet can be very easily turned into a cooked diet.

After two years in remission, Bullet developed a heart condition. To play it safe, I fed him a cooked version of the same diet. I boiled, baked or broiled all of the meat lightly and I steamed the vegetables. Once Bullet's cardiac problems were stabilized, and with his approval, I switched back to his raw diet.

The oils in a cancer diet that provide Omega 3 fatty acids should never be heated—they can be added into the mixture and frozen, or they can be added to individual meals as they are served.

If you cook meat for your dog, cook it in water and save the "gravy" produced in the process. Freeze it in containers and then thaw as needed to pour over your dog's meals. After thawing, dispose of solidified fats that will congeal at the top.

## How Hard Can It Be?

Preparing food for a dog is not as difficult or as time-consuming as you might think. Granted, it's more involved than pouring kibble into a bowl but it is, in fact, pretty simple. On the following pages, you'll find a cookbook-type guide to my routine for preparing His Highness' food and an ingredients list on page 79. Follow it as closely or as loosely as you like.

An excellent diet for cancer dogs that approximates a homemade version of n/d can be found online at [www.veterinarypartner.com]. At the main web page, type into the search box: "Susan Wynn" and click "Search." If this fails, just type the name into your favorite search engine.

If you change your dog's diet in any way, do so gradually. This applies regardless of whether you are switching from store-bought food to n/d, from kibble to home cooked or from home cooked to

## BULLET'S CANCER DIET INGREDIENTS

Quantities are for one week of fine dining for a 75-pound dog. Proportions are about $3/4$ meat, $1/4$ vegetables, then other ingredients are added. At feeding time, I often mixed in a scoop of Hill's n/d so that Bullet would be familiar with the taste.

Meat may be raw or cooked; vegetables may be steamed or pulverized. Use organic foods whenever possible and *always* give a cancer dog filtered water.

\* Note: Bullet was an "easy keep." He required less food than average to maintain his weight and health. Portion sizes will vary from dog to dog.

### INGREDIENTS

Beef, chicken or turkey..............................3 pounds
Tomatoes ..........................................................2
Cabbage................................................$1/4$ head
Broccoli floret, some stem........................................2
Eggs (yolks raw, whites cooked).........................3
Tofu .................................................................$1/4$ lb
Salmon oil; Cod liver oil; Flax Seed oil: .....6 Tbs
Hulled or cracked Flax Seeds.........................1 Tbs
Garlic ........................................................3-4 cloves

### TREATS

Frozen Whiting or Pollack fillet .............1-2/day
(Frozen Smelts can be substituted for small dogs)
Frozen-then-thawed RAW chicken wing ..............1/day
Plain organic yogurt...............................1 small bowl/day
Chopped up broccoli or string beans............on demand
"Cheese bone" ......................................................1/day
(Press cheese into a hollow beef bone; dishwasher-safe)
Raw frozen beef bone with marrow .........................1/day

raw. Mix the new diet with the old, $1/4$ to $3/4$, for a week. Continue to increase the new and decrease the old by $1/4$ each week. At the end of the month, you can donate any remaining "pre-cancer" food to your local shelter.

# BULLET'S PRE-CANCER DIET

Bullet's cancer diet can be revised for a healthy dog. In families with more than one dog, this is helpful because you can prepare Bullet's Cancer Diet for your dog with cancer and at the same time, prepare food for your dog or dogs without cancer.

The non-cancer diet contains less oils and more carbohydrates (e.g., brown rice, potato, oatmeal, quinoa, etc.) than does the cancer diet. Carbohydrates have fallen out of favor in human diets and pet foods as well. They are a source of energy, however, are contained in fruits and vegetables, and carbohydrates do play a role a healthy diet. Additionally, feeding a dog an all-meat diet may be too much protein for your dog and may be too expensive for you to support!

Before Bullet was diagnosed, I fed him meat, whole grains and vegetables, proportioned at one-third each. If you have a cancer dog *and* a healthy dog, you could serve the same food to both, but add cooked rice or other carbohydrates to one of the dishes at serving time.

To prepare a diet to feed to a dog with cancer and also to a healthy dog, prepare Bullet's Cancer Diet without the oils and freeze portions. At feeding time, add carbs to the dish for the dog without cancer, and add oils to the dish of the dog with cancer. Both can have some oils (Omega 3 fatty acids), but give the dog with cancer a double dose.

# About Bullet's Cancer Diet

Once a month, I purchased ten to twelve pounds of organic beef and then spent a couple of hours preparing it. I bought any cut that the butcher was willing to discount, generally in slabs but occasionally ground. Bacteria contaminate ground beef much more quickly than unground, so if you use ground beef, it's important to purchase, prepare and freeze it as soon as possible.

My recipe was never the same from one month to the next. I always included beef, chicken or turkey; flax seed, salmon and/or cod liver oils; broccoli, tomatoes and cabbage; eggs, tofu and garlic. I sometimes included brussels sprouts, broccoli sprouts, beef liver, beets and/or carrots.

After mixing the ingredients, I scooped the food into freezer-bags or containers and placed these in the freezer. During the month, I thawed one bag in the refrigerator and when Bullet ate the last meal from that bag, I rotated another down from the freezer to the refrigerator.

A one-month volume of food for Bullet would have required more containers than I owned and would have occupied more freezer space than I was willing to give up, so I packed the food in freezer bags. When I prepared a smaller volume of food—say a week's worth—I used plastic or glass freezer containers.

When my schedule didn't allow for the full preparation routine, I prepared the diet piece meal. I combined the meat and oils in containers and froze these. When I had time, I prepared the veggies-plus ingredients in other containers and froze these. At meal time, I combined the two components. The only difference was serving from two containers of thawed food instead of just one.

Bullet had virtually no carbohydrates in his diet for two solid years, with the exception of the pound-cake-and-pills combo, two dog biscuits daily and the carbohydrate content in low-sugar vegetables. He had no grains, pasta, potatoes, bread, cereal or other foods that contain high levels of sugar or starch.

I honestly didn't think Bullet would live long enough to suffer negative consequences of a carbohydrate-deficient diet. Once he lived that long and longer, I reintroduced carbs into his diet and he absolutely devoured them, as though on some level he knew he'd been deprived of carbohydrates. Every night before bed, we each had a bowl of oatmeal and I often added brown rice to his meals as well.

# WATER

A dog in cancer treatment may experience vomiting and/or diarrhea. Either, if extended or severe, can lead to dehydration. Monitor your dog's water intake and periodically check for dehydration (see page 65, bottom left). Call your veterinarian if you suspect that he is dehydrated.

When Bullet was diagnosed with cancer, a woman told me that although eating organic food and drinking filtered water may not be necessary for everyone, these are essential components of beating cancer. I was skeptical at the time but her words have stayed with me and now, years later, ring true.

In most areas of the country, tap water is shown in periodic studies to be potable, or safe to drink, with acceptable levels of toxins. "Allowable" levels of impurities in water may be tolerated by a dog or person with a healthy immune system, but for a cancer patient, filtered water is a must.

The simplest method of providing your dog with filtered water is to purchase a countertop filter and place it right over your dog's water bowl. Just open the spigot and fill the bowl. This is the most economical way of providing filtered water.

A more sophisticated (and expensive) method involves the installation of a whole-house water filter. A state of the art system would also include a reverse-osmosis filter that feeds into a separate spout at the kitchen sink. If you're considering

---

## LEADING A DOG TO... MEAT-JELLO!

*Michael Penney's dog, Hobbes, was diagnosed with lymphoma in August of 2003. Michael discovered the following method of increasing Hobbes' fluid intake.*

▸ Mix gelatin (or pectin) with water per directions
▸ Boil lean beef, chicken or turkey in a small amount of water to make a concentrated broth
▸ Add broth to gelatin and let cool
▸ Pour into ice cube trays and place trays in the freezer

Your dog may eat the solidly frozen cubes right out of freezer, or may prefer to let them thaw and drink the liquid. Meat-Jello helped to get Hobbes to drink when he was reluctant to, and provided a bit of nutrition as well.

Printed by permission of Michael E. Penney, Holliston, MA.

---

installing a water-filtration system for your pup, plug into the "pro" column the fact that the whole family will benefit! For homeowners, a good filtration system is also a good investment and will be an attractive asset when you resell your house.

If your dog is dehydrated due to vomiting or diarrhea, or if you feel he's not drinking enough fluid, try Michael Penney's solution to this problem in "Leading a Dog to Meat-Jello," on page 81.

# FEEDING FROZEN

When a dog in cancer treatment stops eating, there is cause for concern. Reversing the "not eating" state of affairs is of the utmost importance even, if necessary, at the expense of breaking the cancer-diet rules. If your dog will not eat the foods recommended for cancer patients, get him to eat foods that are not recommended. Try deli-meat, baby food, cat food, oatmeal...try anything and everything until you find the thing that he will eat.

### FROZEN FISHIES

During Bullet's first "flat out" episode, he stopped eating and showed no interest in food. He'd always been a chunky guy, so I didn't panic at first. I checked his temperature, which was well within the normal range for a canine at 101.5

degrees Fahrenheit. I concluded that Bullet was nauseous—a common chemotherapy side effect. I gave him anti-nausea supplements and remedies with no result.

After several days passed and Bullet had not eaten anything at all, I became alarmed. I was now determined to get him to eat. I held bits of meat to his lips, trying to push the limp things into his mouth with no success. I tried warming up the food, but he turned his head as though nauseated. After many attempts, I finally found success.

Siberian Huskies are Northern dogs, sled dogs, happy eaters of frozen seal meat and the like. This mental image, combined with the realization that frozen food has little or no taste or smell and thus might be more palatable to a nauseous dog, prompted me to attempt the following.

I bought a bag of frozen smelt. I withdrew one and held its pointed tail in the corner of Bullet's mouth, poised to give a gentle push when his jaws opened. I applied only gentle pressure...and waited. Eventually, Bullet's jaws opened slightly and I pushed gently and waited. Lo and behold, just when my fingers were about to become completely numb, a chewing reaction began!

For a few days, I periodically offered Bullet food in a bowl or out of my hand. When it became clear that he was not planning to eat on his own,

I resorted to the "Frozen Fishie" method. After perhaps a week, when his gastrointestinal chemotherapy side effects diminished, the not-eating came to an end and Bullet returned to his normal eating habits.

If your dog isn't eating and you use the Frozen Fishie method, be patient and get comfortable! It may take some time for his chewing reaction to kick in. If he tries to push the fish out of his mouth with his tongue, gently replace it in the corner of his mouth. He may become ticked off at your efforts—in this case, of course, stop trying. We hope that he will instead become tired of pushing it out and let it rest there. Eventually, you will see a reflexive chewing action begin.

"Frozen Fishies" saved the day many times during Bullet's cancer treatment. After his appetite returned, he continued to eat Frozen Fishies. I bought bags of Whiting and Pollack fillets (labeled "dressed" fillets) in the frozen fish section of the supermarket. These are not breaded and there's no sauce—just plain fish meat sans head, skin and bones, ready to serve up raw-frozen, raw-thawed or cooked. Bullet ate a Frozen Fishie every single day from that time forward. I would toss a fish straight from the freezer onto the porch and Bullet would run after it, bark at it, toss it in the air and eventually consume it happily.

If your dog likes frozen fishies, I predict you will have great fun with them. Toss a fillet straight from the freezer onto the porch or into the pen. No dishes to clean, nothing to mix, no muss, no fuss! So long as your dog eats the fillet while it's still frozen, there will be no fish residue or odor on the floor. Not so, however, for his breath! If you like to give your dog kisses, I recommend that you wait a while after he eats his fish, or give his teeth a good brushing before your next smooch.

## VARIETY FOR LIFE

There isn't any one food or combination of foods that you can feed your dog every time he eats, and be confident that you're giving him the best foods to fight cancer. Flexibility, variety and rotation are important.

The most important benefit of feeding your dog a homemade diet rather than processed food is that he will be eating whole foods. An added benefit is that it's easy to provide variety.

The twelve pounds of beef that I bought every month lasted about three weeks. Beef was the mainstay of Bullet's Cancer Diet, but for the last few days of each month, I substituted chicken or turkey; occasionally lamb or venison. I often cooked up a bag of the same Whiting fillets that he ate raw-frozen every night as a snack. When Salmon steaks or fillets were on sale, I used that as the "meat" portion of the meal. Tina Aiken, DVM, at Pine Plains Veterinary Hospital in Pine Plains, NY recommended that I also include organ meat and ground bone in his diet.

The core vegetables in Bullet's diet were those that are high in vitamin C, low in sugar content, and considered to be important in an anticancer diet. They include tomatoes, broccoli and cabbage. Other vegetables high in Vitamin C can also be used. Include broccoli sprouts and any cabbage-family member (such as brussels sprouts or bok choy), kale, spinach, cauliflower, red peppers and garlic cloves. Use carrots and beets sparingly due to their high sugar content.

Pumpkin squash is beneficial to human cancer patients and pumpkin in particular is a remedy for diarrhea. Grapes also may benefit people with cancer, but should *not* be fed to dogs. Grapes and raisins are currently thought to be toxic to dogs. Before it was known that they were toxic, I did include grapes in Bullet's diet and he had no ill effects. I know many people, including a few veterinarians, who give their dogs grapes with no negative results. Still, there are warnings against giving grapes to dogs, so I recommend that you do not include them.

# DON'T FORGET THE TREATS!

Most commercially produced dog treats are high in carbohydrates and are not on the "approved" list for our cancer dogs' consumption. Still, our cancer pups should certainly not be deprived of yummies! Quality of life includes being rewarded for good behavior and, in my book, survival is very good behavior indeed! We simply need to be creative in finding treats that are good for our pups fighting cancer.

Try these cancer-healthy treats on your dog. If he isn't interested, be creative. Try anything he might like that doesn't contain sugar or starch.

### TREATS

- ▸ Plain organic yogurt
- ▸ Cooked turkey or chicken meat, diced
- ▸ Raw, chopped vegetables. Try broccoli, string beans or carrots. Especially good for dogs who like crunchy treats. (Remember, not too many carrots because of the high sugar content.)
- ▸ "Cheese bones." These are easy to prepare. Just press a slice of cheese into the end of a hollowed out, marrowless beef bone. A cheese bone will keep a dog busy for a while, is refillable and dishwasher-safe.
- ▸ Frozen treats - see next section.

### FROZEN TREATS

Bullet loved all of the following treats, and he ate them raw-frozen. Those marked "MUST be raw!" can have very serious or fatal consequences if served after being cooked. *Never* give a cooked bone to a dog!

▸ Hill's n/d (slide out of can, cube and freeze)

▸ Whiting or Pollack fillets; smelts

▸ Chicken hearts

▸ Beef bones (soup bones)—MUST be raw!

▸ Whole chicken wings—MUST be raw!

▸ Turkey necks—MUST be raw!

The items in this list that aren't followed by the note: "Must be raw," can be served cooked or frozen... but if cooked, they seem more like food items than treats, don't they?

Give Bullet's Frozen Fishies a try with your dog. They're the best dog treat ever, bar none. They are extremely healthy, they're simple and fun and most dogs love them. They even get the back of a dog's teeth clean, where most of us don't manage to reach with the toothbrush. Frozen Fishies provide exercise for your dog's teeth and jaws! They are simply the perfect dog treat.

See if your dog loves Bullet's Frozen Fishies as much as Bullet did. If he eats them immediately, you've got a winner. If not, you can cook them up for your own dinner!

*Notes*

# WHAT ELSE CAN I DO? 8

*Do anything and everything*
*And when there's nothing left to do*
*Give a kiss and*
*Sing a song*

You've decided on a medical plan, you're putting together a team of advisors and you have put a cancer diet into action. Now you're asking, *"What else can I do?"* It's time to add supplements to the home-care regimen.

Many supplements can be used in addition to or in some cases instead of traditional cancer treatment. Some natural remedies may protect your dog from the various ravages of chemotherapy, radiation or surgery.

Supplements claiming to fight cancer are, for the most part, untested. Your selection process will therefore be largely guesswork. Many veteran caretakers of cancer dogs, holistic veterinarians and, of course, vendors believe that supplements play a crucial role in the fight against cancer. Many traditional veterinarians and some veteran cancer-dog caretakers say with equal certainty that few or none of the supplements that claim to fight cancer are effective.

Marlene Hauck, DVM, PhD, Assistant Professor, Oncology at North Carolina State University College of Veterinary Medicine, treats Buddy. This yellow Labrador Retriever appeared at the ACVIM's 21st annual Forum in 2003. At that time he was 9$^1$/$_2$ years old and had maintained a 6-year remission from lymphoma. In March 2004, Dr. Hauck was kind enough to answer a few of my questions about Buddy, as follows. (Dr. Hauck's responses are printed in italics.)

AN INTERVIEW WITH DR. HAUCK

What chemotherapy protocol and what other medical treatment was Buddy given?

*Buddy received standard of care chemotherapy with a multi-agent, doxorubicin-based protocol. When he developed cardiotoxicity, the doxorubicin was changed to mitoxantrone. He received appropriate treatment for his cardiac disease as recommended by our cardiologists.*

Did Buddy ever come out of remission?

*Yes, he has come out of remission once so far.*

Can you offer a hypothesis explaining Buddy's (and other survivors') very long survival of canine lymphoma?

*Tumor heterogeneity. While we have prognostic factors for groups of animals, we cannot predict, at this time, how an individual patient will respond to treatment.*

What sort of diet was Buddy fed?

*Normal dog food. At one point, we considered putting him on a special diet for his heart, but I don't think we did so.*

What supplements or alternative treatments did you or Buddy's owners provide?

*Buddy did not receive any supplements or alternative treatments.*

Is Buddy still alive?

*Yes, Buddy is still alive.*

Most veterinary oncologists that I've spoken to do not recommend "anticancer" supplements for their canine patients. According to Robert C. Rosenthal, DVM, PhD, diplomate ACVIM, diplomate ACVR,

*Many owners are interested in complementary or alternative treatments, but none of these approaches have been shown to be of benefit for dogs with lymphoma. It is likely, but not a certainty, that most of these treatments will be innocuous.*[1]

## TO SUPPLEMENT OR NOT

Despite Buddy's longevity *without* the benefit of dietary and supplemental therapies, most of the cancer-dog caretakers I've interviewed want to cover all the bases just in case the supplements actually do give their dogs a better chance at survival. This is not a simple task. There's an endless list of pills, gel caps, capsules, powders, tinctures and teas that claim to fight or cure cancer. If you research in this area at all, you'll hear and read about many alternative treatments for cancer.

Give each due consideration but realize that no one has ever done *everything* that can be done for a cancer dog. It's simply not possible to provide every medical treatment, every supplement and every alternative treatment. As the caretaker of a cancer dog, you must draw the line where you need to and where it makes sense for you.

Choose alternative therapies carefully. Those that have not been scientifically, methodically tested in a controlled environment may or may not be effective. Some that seem to have merit may be worth adding if they're not too expensive and have been found not to have side effects or interfere with traditional treatment.

Remember to be fluid and flexible in your choices of supplements so that you can do each day what's best for your dog according to his current status and needs. From time to time, you might want to add in a new supplement and/or omit one that, in your mind, is less likely to be helping your dog fight cancer.

Few supplements, if any, have been sufficiently tested to inspire any certainty of efficacy. The lack of testing is in large part due to the astronomical costs involved in performing the

## DECISIONS YOU CAN MAKE

▶ **Consultants:** Choose your team members by referral or reputation and revise at will. The only goal is to have the strongest team possible.

▶ **Tests:** You have a great deal of say-so when it comes to testing. You can decline a test based on your dog's comfort level and the benefit to be gained by having the test. Gather information and consult with your team—the final decision is yours.

▶ **Leave or Wait:** If being left at the veterinarian's office is stressful for your dog, wait for the procedure and take him with you whenever possible. Remember, no one wants to be in a hospital longer than necessary—dogs included.

▶ **Shaving:** It's often necessary to shave some fur before surgery or chemotherapy, but generally not for a blood test. It's easier and quicker for the veterinarian but most will make the extra effort to draw blood without shaving if you so request.

Make every attempt to keep your dog intact and beautiful during treatment. It's easy to wind up with a patchwork dog, so keep the shaving to a minimum from the start.

You can specify which leg should be used for testing and treatment. If, for example, your dog is favoring a leg, you can request that a different leg be used for treatment.

▶ **Revisions:** If your dog isn't able to tolerate a treatment, ask your team members to suggest other options. There may well be another treatment that's equally effective and that your dog can better tolerate. If your dog is very ill, consider postponing the next treatment until he's stronger.

You're not at the mercy of any prescribed treatments, medications or schedules, but stick to the plan unless there's a reason to revise it.

extensive testing required for FDA approval. Not many manufacturers of alternative health products can finance the testing and approval process.

Some testing has been conducted for many of the supplements, but on a smaller scale or without the controls necessary to qualify as FDA-level testing. The test population may be too small, dosages and frequencies not adequately controlled and/or the testing is not conducted as a double-blind test.

There is a great deal of anecdotal information about the success of various cancer fighting formulations. Most are documented by physicians, veterinarians or people who have used the product. Many manufacturers will provide a list of testimonials from users of the product, either on their web sites or in pamphlets.

The following section contains an overview of supplements commonly recommended for cancer dogs. This is not a comprehensive listing by any means. Consult your veterinary oncologist, your holistic veterinarian and/or your health store advisor to establish which supplements to give your dog and in what amounts.

## SLOW DOWN

There is an endless list of supplements that allegedly fight cancer. Some are known to offer benefits to the cancer patient and others are thought to help. You might be inclined to use all of them: Don't! You'll spend a great deal of money, become overwhelmed and traumatize your dog with constant pilling. Use restraint and discrimination and select 5 to 10 supplements to start out—choose the ones that you believe will be effective—then revise the list as needed.

Many dogs become reluctant to eat when they're ill, whether the illness if due to cancer,

---

### DON'T BLOW A FUSE!

In the summer of 2000, my kitchen counter was strewn with medication bottles. Each bottle was wrapped with a strip of masking tape with instructions written on it. BID, TID, with food, orally alone. TID 2 days before chemo to 2 days after, BID not before or after chemo...

I'd venture into the kitchen several times a day, scan the array of bottles, vials and powders and feel overwhelmed. As time went on, a routine developed. I periodically eliminated a supplement and added a new one, keeping the list current and dynamic.

When you set out to develop a treatment plan for your dog with cancer, be realistic. Begin with a few supplements that you believe will be most effective. When you learn from a reliable source of a new supplement that's thought to fight cancer, add it to your list and omit any that have been found not to be effective.

---

chemotherapy or some other, unrelated cause. If your dog is "off his foods" and you are working hard just to get some nutrition and essential medications into him, put aside any supplements that aren't working to heal his immediate condition until he is feeling better. Basic nutrition and the medications known to be effective are far more essential than the supplements that may or may not be effective.

Don't add supplements to your dog's regimen willy-nilly. Apart from the potential for cancer-fighting and immune system boosters to wipe out your savings account, apart from the certainty that you'll blow a fuse trying to keep it all straight (which to give when, how many times a day, with food or without, give only before and after chemotherapy or do not give within "x" days before or after chemotherapy) and apart from the possibility that the supplements you choose won't be effective, there is a more dangerous possibility.

Interactions can occur between supplements or between a supplement and a prescribed medication. Some supplements interfere with the intended activity of certain prescription drugs or chemotherapy agents. Regarding supplements that many cancer-dog caretakers give their dogs, Dr. Rosenthal says, "Reports of adverse reactions are beginning to surface, and clinicians should be aware that there are no good data on possible interactions of the alternative compounds often suggested in varied combinations, either with each other or traditional cytotoxic agents."[2]

Speak to your veterinarian and other cancer dog caretakers. If your veterinarian isn't up to speed on supplements (many are not), find a holistic veterinarian to consult in person or by phone.

After deciding on a list of supplements that you want to include in your anticancer program, comparison-shop for the best prices at a health food store and on the Internet. Some supplement products also vary in quality from one manufacturer to another. Through companies such as Consumerlab.com, LLC, research the relative quality of supplements as produced by various manufacturers.[3]

## VITAMINS AND MINERALS

Vitamins and minerals are fundamental to any dog's diet. When a dog is combating cancer, they are essential. Dr. Messonnier states: "Studies demonstrate that both people and pets with inadequate nutrition cannot metabolize chemotherapy drugs adequately.... This makes proper diet and nutritional supplementation an important part of cancer therapy."[4]

# Immnunonutrition: Using Supplements Sensibly

*by Dr. Alice Villalobos*

In the 35 years that I've been treating dogs with cancer, only recently have I found reason to be concerned about over-supplementation. Two wonderful clients came to see me, each with a list of more than 50 supplements that they give their dogs with cancer.

I admire the quest. I understand why caregivers will grasp at any and all remedies that claim to fight or cure cancer. But take care not to over-stimulate your best friend's immune system.

An over-active immune system is vulnerable to such immune mediated diseases as anemia, inflammatory bowel disease, Lupus, hypothyroidism or Addison's disease. For dogs with lymphoma or leukemia in particular, it's best to select supplements that strengthen the immune system by boosting the production of NK (Natural Killer) cells but do not raise the general white blood cell count.

Provide supplements for your dog under the supervision of a doctor who understands how to balance the immune system of a dog with cancer. Supplements are powerful and can cause harm if not chosen wisely.

Cancer evolves through three basic stages, as follows:

▸ **Initiation:** Exposure to a carcinogen such as sun, tobacco smoke, 2-4 D weed killer, asbestos or virus. This initial exposure may result in permanent damage to DNA but is not a direct cause of cancer.
▸ **Promotion Events:** A promotor (abnormal protein sequence on a gene) overstimulates cell division and results in the formation of tumors. This process is not well understood as yet. When a promotor is in the same tissue that has been exposed to a carcinogen, cancer is likely to result.
▸ **Progression to Malignancy:** The controls that normally govern cell cycle progression are suppressed or malfunctioning, resulting in the uncontrolled proliferation of abnormal immortal cells that have lost their programmed cell death signals. These invade surrounding tissues and spread (metastasize) to other parts of the body.

Some components of supplements and mushrooms may interfere with tumor initiation by acting as antioxidants or by upregulating enzymes involved in the natural metabolic ability to break down and detoxify carcinogens.

Supplements containing compounds from mushrooms (in particular, glycoproteins/ polysaccharides) may be effective at promotion and progression stages by killing tumor cells or by interfering with angiogenesis. These may also discourage the development of new tumors by upregulating tumor-suppressive mechanisms.

The body's inflammatory responses also play a role in certain cancers. Inhibition of inflammation (with dietary Omega 3 fatty acids, fish oils and reducing exposure to irritants, allergens and smoke) may result in inhibition of tumor development and regression of some existing tumors.

The immunonutrition program I use for my canine cancer patients is presented in the article, "Sensible Supplements for Immunonutrition." [www.veterinarypracticenews.com] see Archives, Oncology. In print, see Veterinary Practice News magazine, December 2004, p. 24.

Alice Villalobos, DVM, recipient of the Bustad Companion Animal Veterinarian and UC Davis Alumni Achievement awards. President-elect, American Association of Human-Animal Bond Veterinarians and Director, Animal Oncology Consultation Service, Woodland Hills and Torrance, CA.

After deciding on a list of supplements to give your dog, ask your veterinarian or a veterinary nutritionist to look it over to find any conflicts or cumulative excesses. In 2001, at the recommendation of Dr. Ogilvie, I started giving Bullet Centrum Silver® daily. As a result, his entire supplement list had to be reviewed and revised.

### SOME GENERAL GUIDELINES

▸ Vitamins A, C, D, E, K and beta-carotene are important supplements for cancer patients because of their antioxidant properties.

▸ Vitamin A in combination with beta-carotene may benefit patients undergoing chemotherapy, surgery or radiation for cancer.

▸ Vitamin E is thought to protect against the ill effects of the chemotherapy agent doxorubicin while enhancing its effectiveness. Ask your veterinarian for the proper dosage of this vitamin.

▸ Zinc and Magnesium may be helpful in the fight against cancer.

▸ If your dog is predominantly or fully a particular breed, ask your veterinarian if there are any deficiencies typical to that breed. For example, Huskies tend to be Zinc deficient.

Your dog gets some nutrients through his diet, whether it's a home-prepared diet or a commercially produced dog food. How can you know which nutrients he needs in supplement form, and in what quantities? There is a blood test called a Bio-Nutritional Analysis (BNA), which can be preformed to determine the amount of each mineral and vitamin in a blood sample and to test organ functioning.

After reviewing the results of a BNA test, your veterinarian will advise you of any deficiencies found in your dog's test. You can then take steps to correct the imbalance. Veterinarians who recommend this test—in my experience only holistic veterinarians do—generally offer to provide a compounded supplement formulated especially for your dog according to the test results. There's no point in having a BNA test unless you are prepared to adjust your dog's diet and supplementation according to the results.

### OMEGA 3 FATTY ACIDS

As discussed in Chapter 7, O-3 fatty acids play a role in fighting cancer. These supplements may be considered a part of the diet rather than supplements. If you do not feed your dog Bullet's Cancer Diet, please make sure you include these in your supplement regimen instead.

Note: Dogs in radiation therapy should not be given O-3 fatty acids until treatment is completed.

# SUPPLEMENTS

When you hear about a supplement that piques your interest, read up on it. Talk to veterinarians, other cancer-dog caretakers and people who have used the supplement. Don't forget to search the net. After collecting your data, choose a group of supplements that you believe in. Remember, you can revise this list at any time.

### IMMUNE SYSTEM AND NK CELL BOOSTERS

Some chemotherapy protocols are highly immunosuppressive. There are varying theories about the wisdom of using antioxidants to boost the immune system when medical treatment is designed to suppress it. Discuss this with your veterinarian or veterinary oncologist before you add immune boosters to your dog's regimen.

Many supplements claim to boost NK cell (Natural Killer cell) activity and/or production. NK cells attack other cells that are unwanted invaders, such as cancer cells. When cancer is present and a dog's NK cells are fighting an ever-growing army of cancer cells, the supply of NK cells may be depleted. Any cancer patient will benefit from increased NK cells. Here are some of the high quality immune boosters to include in a home care regimen for a dog with cancer.

▸ **K9-Immunity**™ from Aloha Medicinals: A powerful immunomodulator containing nearly 200 immunomodulator compounds. For discount coupon, see color pages of this book.

▸ **Agaricus Bio,** from AtlasWorldUSA: Enhances activity of macrophages that destroy or delay the proliferation of damaged cells. For discount coupon, see color pages of this book.

▸ **Astragalus:** Available in capsules, tinctures, extracts and ground or sliced root. Boosts the immune system and acts as a natural anti-inflammatory.

▸ **IP-6:** An NK (Natural Killer) cell booster that is formulated from rice, containing inositol hexaphosphate. Some formulas add Maitake and Cat's Claw as well.

### ANTIOXIDANTS

Many vitamins, minerals and herbs benefit cancer dogs because of their antioxidant properties. Antioxidants turn free radicals (cells that are missing one electron) into healthy cells by adding the missing electron. Free radicals are precursors of cancer cells. Free radicals are likely to become cancer cells if they are not converted into healthy cells through the addition of that missing electron.

You might want to consult your veterinary oncologist before giving antioxidants to your dog while he's in cancer treatment. Some studies indicate that supplementation with a very high level of antioxidants may actually be counterproductive—that it may actually help cancer cells to multiply.

Other studies show that antioxidants are not only safe, but are beneficial to dogs in chemotherapy. Some antioxidants are said to enhance the effects of certain chemotherapy drugs. Having a holistic veterinarian on your team is the best way to ensure that your dog is on the best antioxidant supplements in light of his medical treatment, other supplements and nutritional intake.

Many antioxidants have curative or protective effects on a particular organ or system. These are noted for each antioxidant in parentheses.

- **Vitamins** A, C, D, E, K, beta-carotene and selenium.
- **Black Currant:** Anti-inflammatory properties. (Skin)
- **Cordyceps:** Oxygenates the system. *Not to be used before surgery or with anticoagulants. (Lungs)
- **Coenzyme Q$_{10}$:** Can cause nausea at high doses. (Heart function; gum health)
- **Curcumin** (found in Turmeric): Anti-inflammatory properties. (Heart function)
- **Germanium Sisquioxide:** Oxygenates and

dehydrogenates the body. Give on alternate weeks—one week on; one week off, etc.

- **Glutathione:** An amino acid. Reduces damage to kidneys if used with chemotherapy agent cisplatin. Minimizes diarrhea when used with radiation therapy. (Immune system)
- **Green Tea extract:** Protects against effects of radiation exposure.
- **Hawthorne:** (Heart function)
- **Pycnogenol:** A mixture of bioflavonoids that may enhance the effects of vitamin C as an antioxidant. (Heart function)
- **Quercetin:** An antioxidant bioflavonoid. May enhance the effect of chemotherapy, radiation therapy and hyperthermia. (Allergies; asthma)

"CANCER FORMULAS"

- **Artemisinin:** A Chinese herb that has killed cancer cells in a test tube.
- **Poly-MVA™ (POLYDOX):** A palladium lipoic complex (LaPd) and DNA reductase. Replenishes nutrients that may be depleted during chemo- and radiation therapy. May also encourage tumor reduction.[6]
- **Transfer Factors:** Stimulate immune system function by enhancing the function of lymphocytes called T-Helper cells.[7] See coupon for Aloha's Transfer Factors!

▸ **Essiac Tea:** Burdock root, Sheep sorrel, Slippery Elm bark and Turkey rhubarb root. Acts as an antitumor antioxidant and immunostimulant.

▸ **Hoxsey's Cancer Formula:** Berberine and other herbs. Cytotoxic, immunostimulating.

▸ **Pau D'Arco** and **Cat's Claw:** Anticancer herbs. Alternate weekly rather than giving both together.

▸ **Seacure:** Biologically hydrolyzed whitefish. A protein supplement with many benefits. May alleviate chemotherapy side effects.

▸ **Vacustatin:** Angiogenesis inhibitor; anti-tumor agents. With PGM (proteoglycan mixture), from Convolvulus Arvensis (bindweed).

### ORGAN SUPPORT

Chemotherapy and radiation are toxic and damaging to body tissues. Toxins travel through the digestive tract, kidney and liver. You can strengthen these organs and systems as follows:

▸ **DIGESTIVE SYSTEM**

**L-Glutamine,** an amino acid, supports protein synthesis, improves gastrointestinal repair and regeneration and augments systemic and gastrointestinal immune responses.[8] Perhaps the most important supplement to give a dog in chemotherapy, to protect his GI tract from damage. Protects nerves and other systems.

*\*Do not give your dog L-Glutamine if he has epilepsy or is taking antiseizure medication.*

**Acidophilus** and **bifidus:** good bacteria in the stomach that can be destroyed by chemotherapy. Give as a supplement or add organic yogurt with active cultures to your dog's diet. **Psyllium** husks powder cleanses the colon.

▸ **KIDNEYS**

Digestive enzymes such as **Prozyme**® or **Wobenzym N**® (A digestive enzyme and metabolic anti-inflammatory); **Vitamin C.**

▸ **LIVER**

**Milk Thistle** detoxifies the liver. **SAM-e** is protective. **L-Arginine** is an amino acid helpful in liver disease, heart disease and cancer. It is included in n/d food. If you're not using n/d, provide L-Arginine as a supplement.

### SUPPLEMENTS WITH ANTIBIOTIC PROPERTIES

▸ **Bovine Colostrum,** a substance produced by a cow just prior to the production of mother's milk. Has powerful antibiotic properties. Available in powder or in encapsulated form.

▸ **Echinacea** defends primarily against upper respiratory infections.

▸ **Goldenseal** protects respiratory and digestive systems. This has antibiotic properties and stimulates the immune system.

# ALTERNATIVE THERAPIES

In addition to supplements that can be given to a dog to help in his fight against cancer, there are alternative therapies that may also help.

### ACUPUNCTURE

Acupuncture does not cure or treat cancer, but can alleviate side effects during cancer treatment, supports organs in need of fortification and generally balances body systems and energy flow.

Rodney Page, DVM, diplomate ACVIM (Internal Medicine; Oncology), is the director of the Sprecher Institute for Comparative Cancer Research at the College of Veterinary Medicine at Cornell University. Dr. Page says, "Of the current alternative therapies, I believe acupuncture has the most solid evidence of benefit for the relief of neurogenic or orthopedic pain developing from cancer."

### MASSAGE

If your dog enjoys massage (and who doesn't?), go for it! It will soothe him and will be a time for bonding. It may encourage circulation and healing and will allow you to discover new lumps or bumps early. When massaging a dog with cancer, some say that hand movements should travel away from the heart.

### SYNCHRONIZED BREATHING

If your dog's breathing is labored, shallow or uneven, lay next to him (the spoon position works well). Synchronize your breathing to his and then very gradually shift your breathing to a deep, even pattern. You may hear your dog's breathing shift, trying to stay in time with yours. When you hear a deep, slow breath, a heavy sigh, a cleansing breath, your mission is accomplished.

### OTHER THERAPIES

Myofascial release, Tellington Touch, Reiki and other healing-touch techniques may encourage healing, circulation and relaxation.

# BULLET'S SUPPLEMENTS

Shortly after Bullet's diagnosis, I left an appointment with a holistic veterinarian with a bag full of bottles, vials and boxes and with very little understanding of what they were or how they worked.

As I gathered knowledge about the supplements, I fine-tuned his regimen many times. The supplements that I consider to be most important for a cancer dog (in addition to E, C, B complex and a multi) are named below. If you use these, please discover correct quantities for your dog.

▸ **Astragalus:** I found dried astragalus root at an herbalist's shop. Slices of the root resemble tongue depressors, and can be steeped in soup, stew or in a cup of tea. One day, a slice fell to the floor on its way to my teacup, and Bullet attacked it! He tossed it in the air, chased it and devoured it entirely. Crunch, crunch. I added it to my list of Bullet's treats, and also often sprinkled a three-finger pinch of shredded astragalus root onto his meals.

At times, Bullet ate astragalus eagerly and at other times showed no interest. According to my herbalist, he was self-medicating. He ate it when his system required it.

▸ **Antioxidants:** Cordyceps, $CoQ_{10}$, Germanium, Quercetin, Pycnogenol... (see list on page 95). I gave Bullet two or three different antioxidants at a time, in rotation. When I ran out of one, I incorporated a different one into his home care regimen in its place. (Also Vitamins C and E).

▸ **Bovine Colostrum:** I gave this to Bullet as needed, whenever he had diarrhea and particularly when his stools contained blood.

This is a natural antibiotic with many additional immune boosting benefits. It is collected in the first six hours after calving.

▸ **Cancer Formula:** I rotated a variety of herbal concoctions claiming to fight cancer. Some of these were store-bought and others were prepared by my herbalist. Again, I attempted to cover all of the bases.

▸ **IP-6:** About 800 mg twice a day. Bullet started his fight against cancer taking IP-6. I replaced it with MGN-3®, another NK cell booster. MGN-3 is no longer available. *Please read page 92 about over-stimulating the immune system.

▸ **L-Arginine:** 500 mg twice a day. This is thought to be an essential in fighting cancer. It is present in n/d Prescription Diet and if Bullet had been eating that dog food, I would have provided less L-Arginine in supplement form.

▸ **L-Glutamine:** In my opinion this is the most important supplement for any dog having chemotherapy treatment. I prefer the powdered version. It tastes slightly sweet and packing it in a capsule is unnecessary. I gave Bullet 1 tsp of L-Glutamine twice daily throughout his cancer treatment. I doubled the dose a few days before chemotherapy and for several days after. When he had any digestive or excretory problems, I tripled the dose.

‣ **Milk Thistle:** ¼ tsp twice a day starting several days after treatment, for about three days. My herbalist sent wild-crafted milk thistle seeds to be ground in my coffee grinder and added to Bullet's pound-cake-and-pill mix.

‣ **Poly MVA®:** At least 2 ml two or three times a day, up to 4 ml three times a day. I put a few drops on any suspicious lumps and bumps. Poly-MVA can be given intravenously as well.

Veterinary oncologist Gregory Ogilvie administers Poly-MVA for Pets as part of a cancer protocol for dogs. Dr. Ogilvie says, "I am substantially rewarded daily by the many stories of enhanced health and wellness of my patients and the lengthened time the animals have had with their families...and the richness that this incredible relationship brings to their lives."

‣ **Prozyme®:** I gave Bullet about 2 tsp. of this digestive enzyme in his food when he was having nausea, vomiting or diarrhea.

‣ **Wobenzym N®:** A digestive enzyme and metabolic anti-inflammatory. I used this for a short time after Bullet recovered from GI side effects.

# ASSESSING SUCCESS

Please refrain from measuring the quality of care that you provide for your dog according to the number of months or years that he survives. Resist turning longevity and survival times into a competition.

People share success stories about their dogs and they do so with good intentions. They don't realize that hearing these stories can make one whose dog survived only a short time feel as though they failed to perform or to provide adequate care.

Stories about the passing of a cancer dog or treatment failure are not only sad in their own right, but also have the power to fill others with trepidation: *"My dog will go down that road too, sometime soon."*

It's not a race, folks. We do not know how to beat cancer. For those whose dogs survive longer than expected, there's no certainty of what it was that enabled them to survive. Nor do we know why some canine cancer patients don't respond to treatment.

Do your best to fight your dog's cancer, and leave your competitive spirit at the gym!

*Notes*

# WHOLE HEALTH

*The happy play bowing tail wagging pup*
*Who needs brushing and washing and training and play time*
*Doesn't vanish just because cancer cells dwell in his body.*
*Remember ~ health and medical issues are no less likely to occur*
*in a dog with cancer than in a dog without cancer.*

Imagine that your dog survives cancer for six months or a year and your veterinarian finds that his teeth are in need of extensive dentistry. Most dental work requires anesthesia and involves a chance of infection—two things that any dog would be better off without, but particularly a dog who is fighting cancer. It's important to remember that health and medical issues are no less likely to occur to your dog than they are to a dog without cancer.

Keep your dog in tip-top condition while he's fighting cancer. Any neglected health issue can lead to unnecessary complications. Vitamin and mineral deficiencies, for example, can undermine any dog's strength. For a dog with cancer, the repercussions can be more severe and more difficult to resolve.

The emotional upheaval of finding that your dog has cancer, combined with the logistical complexities of providing cancer treatment, can be overwhelming. Depending on the complexity of your dog's cancer treatment and home-care plan, you may have your hands full. Incidentals such as bathing, grooming and brushing his teeth may fall by the wayside.

The home-care tasks directly related to cancer will become routine before long and will require less of your time. Once this occurs, it's very important to reinstate a sound whole health home-care program. Elderly folk quip, "If I knew I was going to live so long, I would have taken better care of myself!" Let's be optimistic and believe that your dog will live long enough, despite cancer, to benefit from your continued attention to his whole health.

During the course of cancer treatment, your dog may be immunosuppressed and, therefore, less able to ward off illness. When any secondary or unrelated health problem arises, find out what the treatment options are. Any veterinarians or specialists that you see should be aware of your dog's cancer status—the standard treatment for a particular illness may not be appropriate for a dog who also has cancer.

If a secondary illness occurs, contact all of your cancer team members to ask their recommendation. Consider all treatment options offered by all factions—allopathic, autopathic, holistic, herbal, homeopathic, naturopathic...and then decide on a course of action. Get copies of all reports and tests to add to your log or journal for future reference.

# WEAK SPOTS WITH CANCER

Be vigilant for certain health problems in your cancer dog. A weekly home-care checkup is the best way to sidestep secondary illnesses and keep your dog healthy and strong during treatment.

### TUMORS

Check your dog's body for tumors regularly. This is very easy to do while you're giving him a massage. If you find any new lumps or bumps, inform your veterinarian.

Just two months after Bullet was diagnosed with lymphoma, Dr. Porzio examined a very small, pink pimple-like growth near Bullet's ear. He said it had the appearance of a benign tumor, and that we should watch it for any increase in size or change in appearance.

The tumor remained unchanged for a year but then suddenly grew to twice its original size. Dr. Hoskins removed it surgically as planned, using a short-acting anesthesia. One year later, another, similar tumor developed at the base of Bullet's ear and was removed. The laboratory report on the excised tissue stated that these were both benign tumors.

### TEETH

When a dog is in cancer treatment, dental hygiene is especially important. Chemotherapy can be destructive to teeth and gums and it's always better not to subject a dog with cancer to dental surgery.

Chewing on bones is good for a dog's teeth. Even so, time will take its toll on tooth enamel and gums just as it does on humans even though we brush twice a day. To avoid traumatic (not to mention expensive) dental cleanings and dental treatments, brush those pearly whites!

Brush your dog's teeth every other day. Be sure to use a toothpaste made for dogs or for human infants—one without any fluoride. A small amount of fluoride is good for our teeth, but it's actually a poison. People are capable of spitting out rather than swallowing, but dogs (and babies) are not. Toothbrushes for dogs are sold at pet-supply stores; a child's toothbrush will work as well. There are toothpastes available for dogs and you can also use toothpastes that are intended for a baby's teeth.

Brushing the fronts of your dog's teeth is sufficient. I know very few dogs good natured enough to allow the inside surfaces of their teeth to be brushed.

If your dog isn't cooperative when you attempt to brush his teeth, introduce him slowly. Settle him down, show him the brush, lift his lip and make one quick stroke across his teeth. Give him a treat immediately. Do this one or more times a day, gradually upping the number of strokes each time. Most dogs become agreeable to the procedure quickly, especially if you find a flavored toothpaste that they like.

Eating frozen food may also be beneficial to a dog's tooth and gum health, although I've seen no research on this subject.

### ELBOWS

Include a check for elbow sores in your routine whole-health checkup—the sores that dogs tend to develop from sleeping on hard surfaces. If you find such a sore, toss area rugs or mats over any hard surfaces on which your dog snoozes. If you suspect that the sores are infected (foul smelling, full of pus or hot to the touch), inform your veterinarian right away.

I doused Bullet's elbow sores with hydrogen peroxide and applied an antibiotic ointment. I then either applied a wrap to prevent him from licking the medicine off, or I applied the medicine immediately before a walk or a feeding.

### NAILS, PADS AND FEET

During chemotherapy, a dog's nails may become brittle and crack easily. Because nails are constantly growing, they are subject to the ill effects of chemotherapy.

In August 2001, Bullet and I were out hiking and I noticed that he was leaving bloody paw prints on the ground. I examined his feet to find that a nail had cracked off very close to its sheath.

Once home, I pushed the open end of the nail into a bar of soap to stop the bleeding. Three more nails cracked off during the following month but then the cracking ended. I increased the egg and tofu content of Bullet's diet to provide more protein, rubbed Musher's Secret® into his nails and pads once a day and kept his nails clipped short.

Since Bullet wasn't hiking and running as he did in his pre-cancer days, the fur between his toes grew long enough to cover the pads. This made for a slippery walking surface, evidenced by Bullet's difficulty in ascending the ramp to the car. Keeping the fur between his toes clipped short gave him better traction.

When a dog has difficulty walking for any reason, clip any fur growing between the toes. This is important after any leg surgery or amputation.

### HAIRCOAT

Because cancer cells divide more frequently than do healthy cells, chemotherapy agents are designed to attack cells that are in the process of dividing. As planned, the agents attack cancer cells, but healthy cells that happen to be in the process of cell division are also targeted.

People in chemotherapy often lose hair because protein-based cells such as hair and nails undergo cell division at a higher rate than do other cells. Most dogs in chemotherapy do not typically lose their "hair" because while the hair-growth pattern in humans is constant, it is seasonal in dogs. Don't forget to keep your dog's coat in good condition by bathing and grooming regularly.

It's common for dogs in chemotherapy to lose their whiskers. Bullet lost all of his whiskers three months after beginning treatment and a few months after his last chemotherapy treatment, new whiskers appeared. These were somewhat scraggly, but Bullet didn't seem to mind.

Eighteen months after beginning treatment, Bullet lost his guard hair coat all at once. My herbalist recommended a supplement called Silica and provided me with dried, ground nettles to sprinkle on his food. The fallout ended but Bullet's guard hair coat never returned. To the end, he had a beautiful coat but shorter, fluffier and softer than the typical Husky coat.

### STRESS AND PILLING

Common sense tells us that stress is not good for a dog with cancer. Watch your dog for signs of stress. Every dog has a different set of stressors, so it's impossible to say just what to watch *for*. Any change in behavior could be an indication that your dog is feeling stressed.

When a dog is ill, pilling can become stressful, especially when there are many pills that are to be given over a long period of time. Putting a handful of medications and supplements down Bullet's throat three times daily would have been stressful for both of us.

▸ **Food-Plus-Meds:** If your dog is eating reliably, mix the pills that are not marked "on an empty stomach" with his food. If your dog is not eating reliably, possibly due to treatment side effects, this method will lead to the disposing of a great deal of uneaten food, along with medications.

▸ **PB&P:** Spread peanut butter or soy butter onto a bit of bread, press the pills into it, then fold it over to make a "Peanut-Butter-and-Pills" sandwich. If your dog is skilled at eating the bread and the spread and spitting out the pills one by one, try another method.

▸ **Pound Cake Plus:** Mix pills and powders in a bowl with a bit of crumbled pound cake. This was our method of choice. Even when Bullet wasn't eating reliably, I could always persuade him to eat the pound cake-plus-meds combo.

An added advantage of using the "pound cake plus" method is that if your dog doesn't eat the offering, it's very easy to pick the pills out and try again later. Once pills have been mixed into a food bowl, they are difficult or impossible to retrieve.

▸ **Mix Powder with Water:** Use a needle-less syringe to mix the powder with filtered water. With a finger on the open end, shake to mix. Place the open end inside your dog's lips and slowly empty the contents into his mouth.

Many supplements are available in powder form rather than encapsulated. If this method works with your dog, buy the powder form when possible.

▸ **Manual Pilling:** There were times when I could not get Bullet to eat the pills no matter what. In these cases, I "pilled him" manually.

### MANUAL PILLING

▸ Stand next to your dog, facing same direction.

▸ With the hand nearest him, reach over his neck and under his chin. Insert your thumb and middle finger between his teeth, on either side of his lower jaw, just to the rear of his "fangs."

▸ Gently but firmly pull down his lower jaw. Use thumb of other hand (holding pills) to lift the upper jaw; insert hand and pills.

▸ Drop pills on his tongue, as far back as you can, and remove all fingers.

▸ Let his mouth close but hold his head up a bit and stroke his neck until he swallows.

The lymphatic system often plays a role in cancer, so it makes sense to avoid irritating the lymph nodes. Dog collars press on the submandibular nodes. Walking harnesses are preferable—for a healthy dog as well—to avoid irritating the nodes and also to prevent tracheal collapse.

Most harnesses cut in behind the front legs, applying pressure to the axillary nodes. I've discovered two lymph node-friendly harnesses: The Hug-a-Dog harness from D3Pet Productions (an open mesh, very cool on hot summer days) and the 3-in-1 Vest Harness from RC Pet Products (see "Resources" for contact information).

# VACCINES AND CANCER

In *Natural Health for Dogs & Cats*, Dr. Pitcairn warns that, "Giving a vaccine to an animal with cancer is like pouring gasoline on a fire."[1] Dr. Dodds reports that a dog's immune system may be compromised by vaccination for up to 45 days and, in the case of rabies vaccine, even longer.

The rabies vaccine is required by law in New York State. Bullet had a 3-year rabies vaccine in October, 1999 and when he was diagnosed with cancer in July, 2000, I didn't think he would outlive the vaccine. In October, 2002 the New York

Dog License renewal form arrived requesting proof of current rabies vaccination. My veterinarian filled out a waiver, which I enclosed with the renewal form and a check. The waiver was accepted without question, and Bullet's license to be a dog was renewed. He had no vaccines at all for his last 4 years and 4 months.

There is a serious risk involved in waiving a vaccine. An unvaccinated dog is at risk for contracting the rabies virus if bitten by an infected animal. If an unvaccinated dog bites a person or another dog, he may have to be tested for the virus. Testing requires the examination brain tissue, after the dog is killed.

A vaccination waiver form is included on page 132. If your dog is due for a vaccine, print this form and bring it to your veterinarian to fill in. Then send it to the state with the form that asks you to provide proof of vaccination.

# OTHER PREVENTIVES

Heartworm preventives and products that protect your dog from flea and tick bites may be problematic for a dog with cancer. Some veterinarians and some owners claim that these products should not be used on a dog with cancer; others claim that they are perfectly safe. There

# VACCINES AND CANINE CANCER PATIENTS

*by Dr. W. Jean Dodds*

Although vaccines are necessary and generally safe and efficacious, they can be ineffective at best and harmful at worst to dogs in selected situations. A vaccine can overwhelm a healthy animal with a genetic predisposition for adverse response to viral challenge. Seemingly healthy dogs harboring latent viral infections may not be able to withstand the additional immunological challenge induced by modified live virus (MLV) vaccines.

Vaccination can overwhelm an immuno-compromised dog. With cancer, the situation is complex because the mere presence of cancer cells can suppress immune function. Cancer-producing viral agents and other chemical carcinogens add to this immune onslaught, leaving the dog at high risk for an adverse reaction to vaccine.

After vaccination with MLV vaccine, a period of viremia begins on the 3$^{rd}$ to 14$^{th}$ day and continues for 2 to 4 weeks. During this period, the immune system activates the dog's cell-mediated response pathways which, in turn, may suppress immune surveillance mechanisms and either permit cancer cell regrowth or aggravate existing cancers.

Currently, about 15 percent of human tumors are known to be caused or enhanced by virus. Viruses also cause a number of tumors in animals and there is no doubt that the number of viruses found to do so will increase as techniques to isolate them improve.

The rising incidence of leukemia and lymphomas in an increasing number of dog breeds is a case in point. T-cell leukemias are associated with retroviral infections. Retroviral infections have also been associated with the production of autoimmunity and immunodeficiency diseases.

Similarly, there has been an increase in the incidence of hemangiosarcomas (malignant tumors of the blood vessel lining cells), primarily in the spleen but also in the heart, liver and skin. They occur most often in middle age or older dogs of medium to large breeds.

The German Shepherd dog is the breed at highest risk for hemangiosarcoma, but other breeds (including the Golden Retriever, Old English Sheepdog, Irish Setter and Vizsla) have shown a significantly increased incidence, especially in certain families. Thus, genetic and environmental influences predispose individual animals to immune dysfunction, which can result in adverse reactions when exposed to vaccines, certain drugs and toxins.

It's tempting to speculate that environmental factors that promote immune suppression or immune dysregulation, including vaccines, can lead to the failure of the immune surveillance mechanisms that protect the body against cancer-causing agents. Also, the cumulative effect of a lifetime of vaccinations may have consequences for a dog in later life, including an increased susceptibility to chronic debilitating diseases.

*W. Jean Dodds, DVM, is president of Hemopet, a nonprofit animal blood bank and greyhound rescue/adoption program that also focuses on clinical research in diagnostic veterinary medicine through its Hemolife division. Dr. Dodds speaks to veterinary and kennel club groups throughout North America and overseas on vaccination issues, autoimmunity (hematology, immunology, thyroid and endocrine disorders) and nutrition.*

are varying opinions on this subject among veterinarians and I have no strong belief in either position.

If you live in an area where heartworm disease, flea infestation or tick bites are not common, you may decide to go without preventive and chance it. Ask your veterinarian how many cases there have been in the past few years.

During the second half of the summer of 2000, after Bullet's diagnosis, I did not apply heartworm preventive or flea and tick repellent. In the summer of 2001, I feared I was pushing my luck and used Frontline® every three months and Interceptor® every month and a half (this was a compromise, since both products recommend more frequent application). In the summer of 2002, I didn't use either. I was afraid to use them and afraid not to. I was compromising—using the preventives every other year—and praying.

When Bullet became ill in November 2002, I feared heartworm. He was coughing and gagging intermittently and I cursed myself for not having used preventive. As it turned out, the cause of the coughing was not heartworm, but heart failure.

It is possible to avoid mainstream preventives, using natural products that may provide protection. Nosodes, for example, may protect a dog against a particular disease. Nosodes formulated

for canine heartworm disease may protect a dog from the disease and can also be given as a remedy when a dog has heartworm disease. Nosodes are homeopathic remedies formulated from the disease itself, as are vaccines. Brewer's yeast (mixed with a dog's food) and a variety of natural sprays also keep fleas and/or ticks at bay.

When vaccines are not given, periodic titer tests are extremely important. Consider titer testing twice a year for any disease against which your dog isn't being vaccinated.

Heartworm disease can be fatal but if detected early, it often can be cured. Lyme disease can be squashed by a course of antibiotics—again, early detection results in the best prognosis. In some cases, the disease persists and can cause long term lameness and/or neurologic symptoms.

Members of the yahoo group "jstsayno2vaccs" use a homemade natural insect repellent with great success and no ill-effects. "Aside from being effective against fleas, ticks and mosquitoes," they say, "our horse and goat people swear by it to keep flies away from them as well!"

### JustSayNoToVaccs recipe

▸ Keep in refrigerator—it will go musty/moldy if left at room temperature. Can usually be refrigerated for 2-3 weeks.

- Pour one quart of boiling water over the following ingredients:
- Rind of one grapefruit, rind of one lemon, rind of one lime, rind of one orange and a handful of fresh rosemary and/or lavender (about a tablespoon of dried herbs).
- Let steep overnight. Strain through cheesecloth and put resulting liquid into mister/spray bottle. Lightly mist yourself and the dogs before outdoor jaunts. Use this repellent several times per day if necessary.

## BE PREPARED

Always be prepared for an emergency. A First-Aid kit might include the following.

### FIRST-AID KIT CONTENTS

- L-Glutamine
- Pepcid AC and elderberry syrup for nausea
- Pepto-Bismol for diarrhea
- Metronidazole (Flagyl®) for mucousy stools. (A prescription drug that is an antibiotic with anti-inflammatory effects.)
- Pain medication—ask your veterinarian to make a recommendation. This is a must for any dog in palliative care.
- Rescue® Remedy, a homeopathic Bach Flower Essence remedy, for stress.
- If you have a large dog, make or buy a gurney-type device that will enable you to transport him to help if he's ever unable to walk.

In my experience and in compliance with Murphy's Law, pets become ill most often on a Sunday or late at night. Locate a 24-hour veterinary clinic nearby. Program the clinic's phone number into your cell phone. Also write or print out directions to keep in your car or wallet. You might want to take a test drive to be sure that you will be able to get there quickly if necessary.

If there is no emergency clinic near you, ask your veterinarian for an emergency phone number so that you can contact him or her for help during the night if necessary.

If you travel, share this information with the person who cares for your dog. Leave instructions with your vet as to who can make emergency decisions about your dog's care in your absence.

When you travel *with* your dog, do a little research before leaving home to locate the nearest veterinary clinic and, if possible, the nearest veterinary oncologist and/or 24-hour clinic. It's a good idea to bring your dog's medical records along to help an unfamiliar veterinarian become familiar with your dog's case quickly.

*Notes*

# FROM WARRIORS TO ANGELS 10

*So Easy to Love; So Hard to Lose*

*The loss of a beloved pet cuts deep*
*When we agree to make the ultimate sacrifice*
*To accept the sadness and pain*
*So that they won't have to*

When does treatment end and palliative care begin? Making this decision may be the hardest thing you'll ever have to do. When do you say, "*The battle against cancer is over, and now we will provide pawspice (hospice) care and maintain a good quality of life for my beloved pet, without pain or suffering, for as long as possible.*"

Some caretakers establish a special bond with their pets. That bond grows stronger over time and deepens whenever the pet requires special attention. Soon after I adopted Bullet, my friend Diane said that each time Bullet would have an illness or injury in the future, our bond would deepen. At the time, I told Diane that I couldn't imagine it becoming stronger.

Every time Bullet had an injury, I recalled Diane's prediction. From July 2000 forward, during Bullet's cancer journey, Diane's words resonated. The Bond did indeed became ever stronger, deeper and more infinite.

During the battle, our dogs are warriors and we are their first lieutenants. We invest time, effort, emotional and physical energy into trying to get more time; into fighting a disease that is outside of our control. The decision to give up the fight invokes feelings of helplessness, guilt and, often, anticipatory grief. In the pawspice phase, we strive not to allow these feelings to distract us from the task of making every moment a good one. We do everything we can to ensure "a good death."

# WHEN PAWSPICE BEGINS

When your dog enters into pawspice care, stop all treatments, therapies and home care modalities that may result in adverse results, but do what you can to delay the decline. Continue exercise, supplements and a healthy diet. Provide all of the things that your dog loves best in life. Take lots of photographs and videos—they will be very valuable when pawspice care ends.

### WHEN DOES PAWSPICE BEGIN?

▸ When treatment is not effective and there are no other treatment options with any promise of success.
▸ When your dog is suffering "too much" from the effects of the disease or of the treatment. This is a judgment call that only you can make. You are the one who can evaluate your dog's quality of life, his level of suffering and his ability to continue the battle.
▸ When you determine that it's time to stop fighting because you, your family or your dog can no longer fight.
▸ Your veterinarian may be the first to suggest that it's time for pawspice to begin. For help making the decision, ask the most compassionate member of your team.

Find out if your veterinarian is available at night or on weekends. If not, try to find a 24-hour clinic near you. Be sure to have pain medication at home, to use in case your dog is suffering.

### DECIDE AND FORGET

Please make preparations, if you haven't already done so. Make these decisions and then forget about them! Get back to providing your dog a beautiful, happy, loving pawspice .

Will your dog be cremated? Find a crematory and write down the phone number, hours, pick-up services, and days of operation. You can choose private cremation (your dog is cremated alone and the cremains that you receive will be only his) or group cremation. The cost difference is significant. Ask when your dog's cremains will be returned to you and in what type of container or urn.

If you prefer a burial, decide where. A pet cemetery? Make the arrangements now. At home? The winter ground is hard in some parts of the country, so if you're planning an at-home burial, prepare a plot in advance and have a casket ready.

During pawspice, try not to grieve. Keep the focus on making these last days or weeks happy ones. Do your best to stay strong for your dog now. There will be more than enough time to grieve later.

Be aware of your dog's quality of life (QOL). There are many factors to consider, including his ability to do the things he loves most, his mobility, and his ability to eat and drink, urinate and defecate.

The most important factor to consider is your dog's degree of pain and suffering. Uncontrollable pain and suffering are clear signs that it is time for pawspice to end; that your Warrior is ready to become an Angel.

### PAIN MANAGEMENT

Pain is the number one factor in QOL. When pawspice begins, start watching for signs of pain, including decreases in: Appetite, activity, social interaction and stamina.

Have pain medicine on hand, at home. Dogs can be given non-steroidal anti-inflammatory drugs (NSAIDs). There are many pharmaceuticals that can help as well. The "Pain Management Guidelines for Dogs and Cats," recently released by the AAHA and AAFP Pain Management Task Force, will help your doctor recommend the best medications to control or manage your dog's pain.

Task Force co-chair Dr. Susan Downing states, "Old age is not a disease. Many of the behaviors we previously attributed to aging are actually driven by pain."

## WHEN PAWSPICE ENDS

During this inevitable phase of pet care, a small word can have a profound emotional effect. Some terms may make you flinch—pay attention and be kind to yourself. Use gentle words that honor your pet and also give you solace.

### VOCABULARY

▸ **The beginning of pawspice**: Instead of calling this the end of treatment or a failure, let's call it the beginning of something.

▸ **The end of pawspice**: A euphemism for that final gift we are empowered to give our pets, to release them from pain.

"Put him to sleep" misrepresents what has happened.

"Put him down" is impersonal; devaluing.

"Euthanasia" is clinical and cold.

▸ **Went to Rainbow Bridge**: A euphemism for death. This fabled place that helps bonded caretakers in grief comes from a beautiful poem attributed to Paul C. Daum. For a beautiful video rendition of the poem, go to [www.indigo.org/rainbowbridge_ver2.html].

"Died" is harsh.

"Passed on" is evasive.

"Transitioned." Well, okay... if you insist.

## WILL I KNOW?

People with pets in pawspice care invariably ask me, *How will I know?* My response is always, *You will know!* I've assured hundreds of people and I can always hear that they are not convinced. They are afraid that they will not make the decision at the right time. Yet, each and every one told me later that I was right—they *did* know.

Trust your connection with and your knowledge of your dog. Trust The Bond. We have the ability and the responsibility to decide when our pets' lives will end. Medical team members and support group members may help by suggesting that the time is near or that the time is now. Their advice is invaluable, but we must ultimately make this decision on our own. Sometime later, we will know that we did right by our friend.

## HOW DOES PAWSPICE END?

We'd all like our pets to die at home, peacefully, in our arms, with no pain. Once in a while, the universe is kind and grants us this wish. It did for Bullet, and I am very grateful for that.

When Bullet went to the Rainbow Bridge on November 20, 2004, I began to revive him but stopped. It occurred to me later that he had had a good death and if I had revived him, the next one might not be so good. I knew that it wouldn't have been a long revival in any case, due to his heart and kidney conditions. I would have to suffer this momentous loss soon.

Often, pawspice ends with euthanasia. Many veterinarians offer at-home euthanasia. The family and dog are relaxed in their own space, with loved ones. Some clinics have a special room for euthanasia, with candles and a CD player so that families can bring special music. Staff members are respectful and do not interrupt, or they attend, to offer the family support. If the doctors at your clinic don't provide an atmosphere of respect and compassion for euthanasia, please educate them.

Even though we know that euthanasia is the right thing to do, it is hard. It is impossible. But we do it anyhow, out of love. Helping a suffering dog get to the Rainbow Bridge is the most important gift we can give. It is the ultimate sacrifice because, at this point, their suffering ends and ours begins.

## EUTHANASIA

In some ways, the loss of a pet is like any loss. Grief is grief. But in other ways, this loss is unlike any other. We have the ability and the responsibility to make treatment decisions and end of life decisions for our pets.

Having the right to make these choices is an *ability* because we are enabled and empowered to make choices that will spare our friends pain and suffering when there is no hope of recovery.

Having this right is a *responsibility*. The word has two meanings, equally relevant. It is a double-edged sword. First, it is our responsibility to make use of our ability, our power, our right, to make this momentous decision on behalf of our pet. But after a caretaker has made that final decision, he is often left feeling *responsible* for having decided that his pet's life should end. Often, we second guess ourselves, question our wisdom, decide in our grief and self loathing that we made a horrible mistake. What an unbearably heavy weight to carry.

At the moment that a dog's pain and suffering ends, the caretaker's begins. It is a choice, an ability and a responsibility, to take on hardship so that our dogs don't have to. It's a sacrifice. It's a gift.

## AFTER THE LOSS

Almost all caretakers experience a deep sense of guilt after the loss of a pet. The responsibility to choose the time rests on our shoulders and it is huge. A sense of urgency is involved in making this decision at exactly the right moment—not too early and not too late. Every day, I speak to caretakers stressing over their ability to decide.

"Too early" means that we deprived our dog of more time and ourselves of more time in his company. A caretaker may suspect or imagine that he ended pawspice too early, but there is absolutely no way to know this for sure. The hope is that euthanasia was performed at just the right time and that otherwise the dog would have suffered. I believe our special connection to our dog informs us when this will happen if we do not act.

"Too late" is more difficult. It means that the dog suffered, and anyone who takes this responsibility to heart does their level best not to wait until the pain has set in. Unfortunately, as you may know from experience, this is not always possible. If your dog experiences pain before you are able to help him to the Rainbow Bridge, remember that the duration of their pain was negligible in comparison to the long, wonderful life that your dog had with you.

In recent years, the position that pets fill in their caretakers' lives has been upgraded. Some of us acknowledge and value our pets as four-legged family members. Others consider the family dog or cat, rabbit, gerbil or ferret to be no more meaningful—and sometimes less valuable—than a piece of furniture. The latter group is not terribly concerned about pet loss and the following does not apply to them.

For the bonded caretaker, after the loss comes the grief. Very often, that grief is tinged with guilt—sometimes terrible guilt, because we are so completely responsible for making that final decisions for our pets. We think, *If only I had made some different choices, my dog would still be here.* In every end-of-pawspice situation, there are things that could have been done differently.

We make the best decisions we can. And then, we must believe that our decisions were the best ones available.

I read many pet loss books when Bullet went to the Bridge. I had to laugh when I found a chapter in one of the books titled: "The Overly Bonded Owner." I suspect the author of that book would include both you and me in that group. That is one group of which I'm very proud to be a member!

# MEASURING GRIEF

You probably have friends and family who are not overly bonded—who don't understand. They complain, *That's enough, it's time to move on!* or *Get over it, he was only a dog!* These comments may be meant to help, but they are insulting and infuriating. If you feel compelled to voice objections and defend yourself—don't! Doing so will only lead to further frustration.

Avoid speaking about your loss to those who do not understand. If you are surrounded by people who don't understand, join an online support group. You are certainly not alone.

### WHAT HELPS
▶ **Find Support**

Do not minimize the effect that your loss has on you emotionally and on all aspects of your life. If you cannot cope with the sadness, please find help.

Attend a pet loss support group. Many shelters and animal hospitals offer them. Your veterinarian may be able to refer you to one.

Often, the group leader is a mental health professional who you can trust to step in if more help is needed. The leader may counsel you privately as well, if you feel this would help.

There are pet loss support groups online as well. My friend Connie lives in a very rural area where there are no pet loss support groups. Connie appealed to a local hospice and was invited with open arms to share her grief in their support group.

If you're more comfortable one-on-one, find a private therapist with experience in bereavement or grief counseling.

▶ **Light Memorial Candles**

When I lost Bullet, I lit a 7-day candle that gave me great solace and comfort. I placed the glass-enclosed pillar candle near the spot where Bullet spent his last days. The flickering flame had a profound effect on me. It symbolized him, his spirit...his presence and his absence. After seven days, when the flame was about to flicker out, I rushed out to the store in a panic, to buy a new one. I just needed to see the flame dancing there for another week.

\* If you light candles in memory of your pet, be sure to position them safely, so that there is no danger of starting a fire.

▶ **Display Photographs and Videos**

Create an album for your dog. Use photographs and any video clips you have, to create a slide show on your computer. You can email your slide show to friends and family, or copy it onto a CD or DVD and mail copies out, in tribute to your sweet dog.

While handling images and remembering the moments they were taken, allow your mind to wander back to the good, happy times captured in each image.

Frame and hang on the wall some of the most special pictures of your dog.

▶ **Hold a Memorial Service**

Gather together the people who knew and loved your dog, for the purpose of paying tribute. Don't forget to invite your veterinarian and clinic staff. They are family too!

There's no "right" time. I had a memorial service for Bullet a month after he went to the Bridge. Twenty people came and we formed a circle around an easel holding a big photograph of Bullet, with his urn beside it. I read the passage on page 129, then Bullet's godfather, Ru Schwager, chanted a prayer. Each person around the circle told a story about Bullet and, finally, we all walked a half-mile trail called Peaceful Path, a trail that Bullet and I had traveled together thousands of times.

▶ **Expression is the Opposite of Depression**

You kept a journal during your dog's illness. Now keep one during the days and weeks after your loss. Write your thoughts and feelings down to document your pet loss journey.

Later, reading this journal, you will revisit the wonderful feeling of your dog having just recently been in your arms. Cling to moments just after the loss, when your dog is still "in the air." His presence will linger in his favorite places, in your head and in your heart.

*Notes*

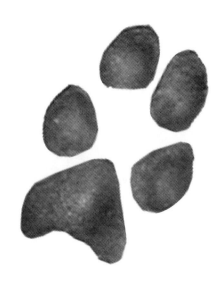

# BULLET'S STORY, PART TWO
## Epilogue

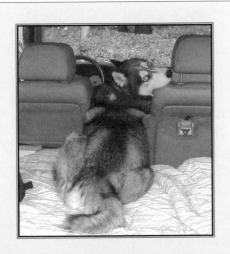

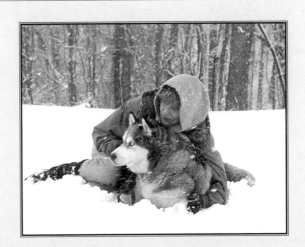

Throughout Bullet's 75-week chemotherapy protocol, I saw him as a cancer dog. My thoughts about him were tinged by the inevitability that at some time—perhaps today or perhaps a year from today—his remission would lapse; he would have chemotherapy side effects; he would slip into cancer cachexia. When someone we love is diagnosed with a terminal illness, our feelings for them are altered. That "someone" may be a cat or a dog just as easily as a human—it can be any living creature that has won our love.

I never took Bullet for granted, but after his diagnosis, my constant vigilance of and concern about his physical health and his quality of life intensified. I didn't think it was possible, but my connection to him became even stronger. After years of remission, I was able to look at Bullet without thoughts of cancer echoing in my head and the bond continued to grow stronger. We had taken a journey together and that journey had changed us forever, individually and as a team.

Bullet began the VELCAP-L chemotherapy protocol on July 18, 2000 and completed it in March 2002. He was 9½ going into chemotherapy, 11 coming out and getting into his senior years. I was truly offended the first time Dr. Hoskins referred to Bully as a "geriatric dog." How dare he! Ironically, I later often referred to Bullet as a geriatric dog with great pride.

During the six months that followed Bullet's last chemotherapy treatment, I saw continual improvement in his health. His posture, his coat quality, eating habits and energy level—even his facial expressions—were once again that of a healthy dog. Once again he was strong, full of energy, playful and happy.

As Bullet regained his willful, playful Husky personality, we fell back into our old routine of arguing over which trail to hike, which toy to toss around, when to get into or out of the car and other very important decisions. He was again able to climb Anthony's Nose, part of the Bear Mountain range, and spend long weekends with his furry friends, running on the beach in Cape Cod.

Bullet was well traveled. I never put him on a plane but he was a wonderful road-trip companion. His self-proclaimed place in my car was sitting with body in the back and chest and paws on the center console. If there were other dogs in the car, they best not attempt to claim this "shotgun" seat of honor. Any attempt to supplant him was met with a demonstration of how he obtained his nickname, "Bullet Growly Bear."

Once settled in, Bullet often rested his head in the crook of my right arm while I was driving. It was perfectly positioned, that head, so that I could easily lean over to kiss it at red lights. Bully often became drowsy and then the full weight of that handsome two-ton head came to rest on my arm.

Apart from our many trips to Cape Cod, our journeys included Lake Placid for sledding when Bullet was young, Washington, D.C. to visit my cousins and Big Indian, NY for long weekends of snow-shoeing in the winter and hiking in the summer. We also took trips to Killington VT, Paoli PA, Oneonta NY, Boston MA and the Delaware Water Gap. Bullet was a great tent camper, always a well-behaved guest at hotels, inns and in the homes of friends.

In November 2002, Bullet developed a cough that sounded just like a cat with fur balls: "*Cough, cough, cough, gaaag.*" Being an experienced cat-caretaker, I was so sure of my "diagnosis" that I gave him hairball remedy for two days. But the cough persisted and off we went to the clinic.

Diagnostic tests revealed that Bullet was in heart failure and was coughing because his lungs were filled with fluid. EKG and ultrasound tests rendered diagnoses of dilated cardiomyopathy and atrial fibrillation. These maladies might or might not have been caused by doxorubicin, a chemotherapy agent used in Bullet's protocol. Doxorubicin is known to cause cardiomyopathy, but generally the damage to the heart is seen closer to treatment and not two years later.

My initial response was that this was an extremely unfair turn of events. Wasn't it enough that my sweet boy had endured cancer and chemotherapy? Then it dawned on me that just because Bullet beat cancer, that didn't earn him immortality! He would, eventually, die from *something*. This was such a simple concept but it somehow took me by surprise.

I was told that if we could get the fluid out of Bullet's lungs and control his heart conditions with medicine, he could survive another six months to a year...or he could die suddenly at any time. I should be prepared for this eventuality.

The medications did clear his lungs of fluid—the same meds that are given to humans with these conditions, just as the chemotherapy agents used to fight canine cancer are pretty much the same as those that treat human cancer. However, after considerable down-dosing, we found that Bullet could not tolerate the one medication that could have reversed atrial fibrillation and allowed a normal heartbeat (digoxin).

I was told many times by many veterinarians over the following two years that Bullet could die at any moment, without warning. I heard this many times and knew it was true, but Bullet and I agreed not to dwell on it. Over the next two years I marveled at Bullet's strength as he just kept plodding along, brushing off all dismal doomsday predictions.

In April, 2003, Bullet had a second left-sided heart failure, with the same coughing symptoms as the first. Dr. Hoskins consulted with a tele-medicine service called Cardiopet and with a cardiologist enlisted via the Advanced Veterinary Care Center in Newburgh, NY to evaluate Bullet's condition . We discussed the options and formulated a plan for adjusting the dosages of Bullet's medications. Once again, his lungs cleared.

In May, 2003, Bullet and I participated in "Dogswalk Against Cancer," an event sponsored by the American Cancer Society to raise funds for cancer research. $2,000 of the money raised at this event was granted to the Cornell University College of Veterinary Medicine. Bullet completed the mile-and-a-half walk in good form.

In August 2003, we visited Margot and Dick Basile, dear friends and proprietors of The China Clipper, a B&B on Cape Cod. Margot and Dick are dog lovers par excellence—complete and proper dog care is a top (if not *the* top) priority in the Basile household. During this visit, Bullet's neck and throat region became so full that he had no neck to speak of. I felt his lymph nodes with trepidation but they were not enlarged. Rather, the area felt mushy and full of fluid.

When I awoke the next morning, Bullet was lying on his side with absolutely no interest in getting up. His belly had become distended and hard overnight and I knew that we were in very serious trouble. The Basiles' veterinarian made a house call to examine Bullet. After a short examination, she directed me to get him to a clinic post haste—a clinic that had an ultrasound unit in-house. Of course, this was a Saturday afternoon.

There ensued a frenzy of phone calls to local veterinary clinics, Dr. Porzio in Canada, Dr. Hoskins in New York and old acquaintances at Tufts Vet School in nearby Massachusetts.

Tracy and I packed up in no time flat and we two, Bullet, Toshi and Kai all piled into the car. During the two-hour drive to the Foster Small Animal Hospital, the 24-hour emergency clinic at Tufts Vet School in North Grafton, MA, Bullet's condition worsened. Bullet stayed overnight at the hospital and Tracy, Toshi, Kai and I found a nearby motel that allowed dogs.

It was congestive heart failure again, but this time both sides of his heart were in failure. Bullet's condition improved marginally overnight, with a nitroglycerine patch on his ear, an injection of lasix and constant monitoring. In the morning, I signed him out "against doctor's advice" to move him to a clinic near home.

After another two-hour white-knuckle car ride with two humans and three dogs, we arrived at the 24-hour emergency animal hospital in Bedford, NY. In response to a "heads up" call by cell phone ten minutes before our arrival, two staff workers were waiting for us in the parking lot with a gurney, ready to transport Bullet from my car into the hospital.

There were diagnostic tests and then revisions in Bullet's cardiac medications. He now had to be given a much higher dose of lasix to prevent his lungs from filling up with fluid and this meant lots of drinking and lots of peeing.

Bullet did recover once again but was not his old spunky self. Dr. Porzio suggested that I look into a cardiac medication for dogs not yet approved for use in the U.S. Via the Internet, I was able to correspond with several people whose dogs had been given this medication in clinical trials and they all claimed that their dogs survived several additional years with good quality of life because of this drug.

Bullet was not eligible to participate in an ongoing clinical trial for this medication because of his history with lymphoma. However, the veterinary cardiologist who gave me this news also explained how to go about getting the drug for Bullet. After finding a pharmacist in Great Britain who was willing to export Vetmedin® (pimobendan), I arranged for the FDA to fax the necessary forms to Dr. Hoskins. A week after he filed these, we had FDA permission to import this wonder drug.

And it was, indeed! Very soon after beginning daily doses of this medication, Bullet's energy level and quality of life improved greatly. He regained his spunk and his "growly bear" -ness. Perhaps my gleeful reaction when he growled and chewed on a friend's hand seemed strange, but to me these were signs that Bullet was himself again.

On March 15, 2004, Bullet turned 13 years old. As always, we were stopped on every outing by passersby with questions about Bullet, stories about other Siberians and great praise for his beauty and grace. *"What's his name?"* and *"How old is he?"* The answer to this last question surprised all. *"But he looks like a pup!"* And I would nod, proudly.

At this time, Bullet was in good form with an excellent quality of life. It seemed we had all of his issues under control. There were episodes of congestive heart failure now and again—five in all—but these were resolved by an adjustment to his dosage of lasix or, if necessary, a lasix injection. Sometimes I thought we could go on like this indefinitely—his cancer and heart conditions were holding steady.

Along with the increased dosage of lasix came increased drinking and increased urination. I looked for a doggie-diaper but found only one and it would require pulling Bullet's tail through a fairly small hole. I didn't even have to attempt this to know that it was not going to work for us.

The diaper holder and diapers worked quite well, but what didn't occur to me until it was too late was that with a diaper on, Bullet wasn't able to clean himself and the area remained constantly wet. In the summer of 2004 there was a heat wave in New York. Because Bullet was indoors (and diapered) all of the time except for quick trips outdoors to relieve himself, he developed a urinary tract infection with bloody urine.

A veterinarian at the emergency clinic extracted a urine sample from Bullet's bladder via a catheter and the infection was diagnosed. After a course of antibiotics, I declined to have his urine extracted via a catheter again or to have a cystosentesis, whereby a needle is inserted through the belly area into the bladder to extract pure urine, uncontaminated by a journey from the bladder through the urinary tract. I opted to provide urine from a "free catch" instead.

The infection remained, but after a course with a different antibiotic and another test from a free catch, the infection was gone. From this point on,

Bullet wore diapers only during certain parts of the day, giving him plenty of time to keep himself clean and to air out.

In May 2004, I discovered a grape-sized tumor on Bullet's side. I immediately stopped feeding him oatmeal and reinstated most of his cancer supplements. A needle biopsy report said that the tumor was most likely malignant. The recommendation: "Removal with wide margins."

"How would you feel," I asked Dr. Hoskins, "about operating on a 13-year-old Husky with lymphoma and heart disease?" He thought about it and said that he felt Bullet was strong enough to tolerate the surgery. Once again, I reached out to Bullet's cancer team members for advice. Unanimously, the consensus was to remove the tumor with wide margins. I scheduled surgery to occur just after the American Cancer Society's 2004 Dogswalk Against Cancer at Bear Mountain.

Bullet was selected as "King of the Dogswalk." Coincidentally, the "Queens of the Dogswalk" were two cancer dogs whose caretakers and I had "met" online at the Delphi forums Pet Cancer Support Group. In May 2004, Bullet, Suzi (Hanon) and Diamond Dreamer (Furstinger) were crowned and admired by all. The royal families then proudly led the procession of people and dogs around Bear Mountain Lake.

The following week, Dr. Hoskins called upon Bullet's cardiac team to recommend anesthesia to be used during surgery. As advised by Dr. Ruslander, the surgery was performed by a board certified surgeon, assisted by Dr. Hoskins.

The tumor was the size of a grape; the tissue removed was the size of a grapefruit. As always, Dr. Hoskins was respectful of my aversion to seeing bare skin on Bullet and was diligent about shaving no more fur than necessary.

Making the decision to have the surgery was easy. In my mind, there was no alternative. Bullet was moving slowly and showing signs of old age, but was still full of personality and enjoying life. When the biopsy report from this surgery described a highly aggressive nerve sheath cancer, it confirmed that aggressive removal had been the right course of action regardless of the outcome.

Bullet did tolerate the surgery. Not surprisingly for a fellow sporting cancer and heart disease at his advanced age, recovery was slow.

In July 2004, *Help Your Dog Fight Cancer* was published and Bullet continued to recover as the book continued to find its way to people who had dogs with cancer. Clearly, it makes no sense to write a book and then hope no one buys it. Still, each order that came through brought sadness. *Another dog with cancer.* But remembering how desperately I had wanted a book like this one four years earlier, each order also makes me glad that I have the book to offer.

By October 2004, Bullet was having difficulty walking. His rear legs were failing and there was little we could do to help apart from surgery, which was out of the question. We went to Cape Cod for what would be our last visit to the Basiles and walked a bit on the beach in the rain. We didn't mind. At this point, Bullet's hind legs were weakening and worsening and so I purchased a wonderful custom-made cart for him from Eddie's Wheels in Shelburne Falls, MA.

In mid-November of 2004, Bullet virtually stopped walking and then stopped eating. A blood test showed that he was in kidney failure and he was dehydrated. I wasn't willing to leave him at the hospital overnight where he might die alone, so an IV catheter was installed in his leg and I set him up in my bedroom with IV fluids. I hoped as always for a recovery, but felt that Bullet might not have any more miracles left.

I prepared a new diet with a lower protein content for his kidneys, put it through a food processor and added water until it had the consistency of a thick soup for force feeding. Force feeding is really just a matter of spooning food into a large tube and then slowly emptying it (by press-ing on the plunger) into the patient's mouth. Bullet was very cooperative about smacking his lips and swallowing a fair amount of food. I gave him water in the same manner, even though he was being hydrated by IV.

On Thursday November 18th, after three days of IV fluids, a blood test showed that Bullet's kidneys had improved. An on-call veterinarian cautioned me not to be optimistic. This test was performed in-house; the previous one at a laboratory; the apparent improvement could be due simply to differing calibrations. He said, *"You don't see kidney values like these in living dogs."*

On the morning of November 20, Dr. Hoskins called to say that Friday's blood test results were back, showing significant improvement. He seemed hopeful that the Magic Bullet might have just one more magic trick left in his bag. Perhaps Bullet really could cheat death just one more time.

Ten minutes later, Bullet died in my arms. I began mouth-to-nose resuscitation but after a minute I stopped. I said, *"Oh, no...wait a minute...maybe I shouldn't be doing this."* I looked down at his sweet face. He was so beautiful lying there as asleep, so peaceful. It shocked and pained me when I realized that I was not going to try to resuscitate him. That I was not going to see him awaken. That he would never again look at me with those beautiful ice blue eyes, not ever again. There were so many treasured things that I knew in that moment would never happen again. Our long, long journey had come to an end And all I could think was *"No, wait, please wait! I'm not finished taking care of you."*

The phone number for the Hartsdale Pet Cemetery and Crematory had been tacked to my bulletin board for four years. I had glanced at it hundreds of times, thinking with a smile, *"I don't need you yet."* Now I made the call and within two hours a young man came to carry Bullet's body gently and respectfully to his station wagon.

The cremation was three days later. Lynn Schwager, my friend and Bullet's guardian in case of my death, was there to support me. We were ushered into a small room to say goodbye and there was Bullet, a bit cold to the touch but he looked and felt just exactly as he did when I last saw him. Lynn said it was amazing how beautiful he was even in death. The following day, I returned to pick up the cremains.

Today, it's been three months since Bullet died. I no longer have to take him outside every two hours. I'm free to go on whole-day outings at will. The constant trips to the vet's office have stopped as have the constant dosings of medications and supplements. And yet, I would gladly and without hesitation give up all of these new-found freedoms for another decade or another minute with Bullet.

I miss his head on my arm in the car, I miss watching my fingers disappear as they stroke his luxurious, deep, soft fur. I miss his cold nose touching my face as a peck more than a kiss. I miss feeling my heart melt when I turn a corner or raise my head from my work to catch him watching me. I miss the stirring, the awe that he elicited, which I can describe only through its likeness to standing at the edge of the Grand Canyon, looking in awe on what nature has made.

I'm grateful that such a remarkable creature graced my life for one shining moment that lasted twelve years, two months and a day.

---

I missed the first 18 months of Bullet's life and I'm grateful that I was given the opportunity to keep him by my side during his twilight years. I'm glad that neither of the beasts—cancer nor heart disease—took him in the end.

This is the story of a very special dog, "The love of my life; The dog of my dreams." It's the story of a shelter dog once named Max who came to be known as Bullet, who earned the titles of Bully, Bullet Growly Bear and King Bully and who will be remembered with love as The Magic Bullet.

# So Easy to Love, So Hard to Lose
# A Eulogy for Bullet

*December 12, 2004*
*Rockefeller State Preserve*
*Sleepy Hollow, NY*

*Thank you for coming to share memories of Bullet, to help me*
*celebrate his life and to say a loving farewell.*

*Bullet and I walked across these stepping stones more than 2,000 times*
*in the 12 years, 2 months and 1 day that he was with me.*
*I can almost see him now, prancing regally, wearing that*
*wonderful Husky smile and lifting each paw high with every step*
*as he moves from stone to stone with the pure and natural grace*
*that can be seen only in a wild creature*
*unaware of and unimpressed by his own beauty.*

*Bullet had a great inner strength—a strength and temerity that enabled him*
*to survive lymphoma. That same indomitable spirit enabled him to survive*
*a heart disease that, two years ago, was expected to kill him within 6 months.*

*There's one thing that Bullet was not—he was not an easy dog.*
*To me, Bullet's willfulness, his wildness, his growliness*
*were all part of his allure.*

*Bullet stole my heart in a split second on September 19, 1992*
*and Bullet will always have my heart. He is my heartdog,*
*the love of my life and the dog of my dreams.*

*He has indeed left pawprints on my heart.*

# REFERENCES

## Chapter 3

1 The Animal Cancer Institute [www.animalcancerinstitute.com/oncology.html]

2 *Small Animal Clinical Oncology,* editors Stephen J. Withrow, DVM, diplomate ACVIM (oncology) and E. Gregory MacEwen, VMD, diplomate ACVIM (oncology and internal medicine). W.B. Saunders Company, 2001, p.233.

3 ibid, p.455.

4 *Animal News,* The Morris Animal Foundation. Volume III, 2001.

5 *Veterinary Oncology Secrets,* editor Robert C. Rosenthal, DVM, PhD. Hanley & Belfus, Inc, 2001, p.180.

6 *Small Animal Clinical Oncology,* p.558.

7 Data for this chart was collected from two sources: *Small Animal Clinical Oncology* and *Manual of Small Animal Internal Medicine,* by Richard W. Nelson, DVM and C. Guillermo Couto, DVM. Mosby, 1999.

8 *Journal of the American Veterinary Medical Association,* April 15, 2004.

9 "Ten Simple Steps to Ecological Lawn Care." *Natural Life Magazine,* May/June 1995, p.2. Available online at: [http://www.life.ca/nl/43/lawn.html].

10 Home Harvest Garden Supply, Inc. (800) 348-4769; [http://homeharvest.com]

11 Peaceful Valley Farm Supply (888) 784-1722; [www.groworganic.com]

12 *Food Pets Die For: Shocking Facts about Pet Food,* by Ann N. Martin. New Sage Press, 2003, p.9.

13 A 2001 report by the American Veterinary Medical Association. Available online at: [www.avma.org/policies/vaccination.htm]

## Chapter 4

1 *Small Animal Clinical Oncology,* editors Stephen J. Withrow, DVM, diplomate ACVIM (oncology) and E. Gregory MacEwen, VMD, diplomate ACVIM (oncology and internal medicine). W.B. Saunders Company, 2001, p.82.

2 *Veterinary Oncology Secrets,* editor Robert C. Rosenthal, DVM, PhD. Hanley & Belfus, Inc, 2001, p.87.

3 ibid, p.90.

4 "Targeting the blood supply of cancer," by Chand Khanna DVM, PhD, Dipl ACVIM (Oncology), 2002. [www. TheAnimalCancerInstitute.com]

5 "Dog's Complete Cancer Cure Opens New Doors In Research," by Erin Kirk. *USA Today,* July 25, 2002.

6 PBS report, March 15, 2007, "Dogs Shed New Light on Cancer Genes in Humans."

## Chapter 5

1 *Manual of Small Animal Internal Medicine,* by Richard W. Nelson, DVM and C. Guillermo Couto, DVM. Mosby, 1999, pp.711-715.

2 *Veterinary Oncology Secrets,* editor Robert C. Rosenthal, DVM, PhD. Hanley & Belfus, Inc, 2001, p.183-4.

# Chapter 6

1   Data for chart collected from:
a)  *Small Animal Clinical Oncology,* editors Stephen J. Withrow, DVM, diplomate ACVIM (oncology) and E. Gregory MacEwen, VMD, diplomate ACVIM (oncology and internal medicine). W.B. Saunders Company, 2001;
b)  *Manual of Small Animal Internal Medicine,* by Richard W. Nelson, DVM and C. Guillermo Couto, DVM. Mosby, 1999;
c)  *Veterinary Oncology Secrets,* editor Robert C. Rosenthal, DVM, PhD. Hanley & Belfus, Inc, 2001;
d)  Monographs for chemotherapy agents; e) Assistance from Dr. Kevin A. Hahn and Dr. Alice Villalobos.

# Chapter 7

1   Science Diet® (800) 445-5777 [www.hillspet.com]
2   Natura Pet Products®, Santa Clara, CA 95052-0271 (408) 261-0770 [www.naturapet.com/].
3   *Natural Health Bible for Dogs & Cats,* by Shawn Messonnier, DVM. Prima Publishing, 2001, p.302.
4   *Veterinary Oncology Secrets,* editor Robert C. Rosenthal, DVM, PhD. Hanley & Belfus, Inc, 2001, p.107.
5   *The Wolf: The Ecology and Behavior of an Endangered Species,* by by L. David Mech. University of Minnesota Press, 1981.

# Chapter 8

1   *Veterinary Oncology Secrets,* editor Robert C. Rosenthal, DVM, PhD. Hanley & Belfus, Inc, 2001, p. 184.
2   ibid, p. 184.
3   www.consumerlab.com
    Phone: (914) 722-9149
4   *Natural Health Bible for Dogs & Cats,* by Shawn Messonnier, DVM. Prima Publishing, 2001, p.45.
5   *Germanium: Its Miracle Healing Effects and Health Implications,* by Yang Hwan Oh. Dorrance Publishing Company, 2003.
6   AMARC Enterprises
    Phone: (866) 765-9682
    Web site: [www.polymva.com]
7   [www.vet4life.com]
8   *Veterinary Oncology Secrets,* p. 107.

# Chapter 9

1   *Dr. Pitcairn's Complete Guide to Natural Health for Dogs & Cats,* by Richard H. Pitcairn, DVM, PhD. St. Martin's Press, 1995, p. 247.

# RESOURCES

## BOOKS

*Beating Cancer with Nutrition*, by Patrick Quillin, PhD, RD, CNS with Noreen Quillin. Nutrition Times Press, Inc., 2001.

*Complete Guide to Natural Health for Dogs & Cats*, by Richard H. Pitcairn, DVM, PhD, and Susan Hubble Pitcairn. St. Martin's Press, 1995.

*Food Pets Die For: Shocking Facts about Pet Food*, by Ann. N. Martin. New Sage Press, 2003.

*Grizz's Story: A Greater Courage*, by Jo Helms. Jo Helms Publishing, 2003.

*Holistic Guide for a Healthy Dog*, by Wendy Volhard and Kerry Brown, DVM. Howell Book House, 2000.

*Home Safe Home: Protecting Yourself and Your Family from Everyday Toxics and Harmful Household Products in the Home*, by Debra Dadd-Redalia and Debra Lynn Dadd. J. P. Tarcher, 1997.

*Kindred Spirits: How the Remarkable Bond Between Humans and Animals Can Change the Way We Live*, by Allen M. Schoen, M.S. D.V.M. Broadway, 2001.

*Natural Health Bible for Dogs & Cats*, by Shawn Messonnier, DVM. Prima Publishing, 2001.

*Natural Nutrition for Dogs and Cats*, by Kymythy R. Schulze, CCN, AHI. Hay House, Inc., 1998.

*Pets Living With Cancer*, by Robin Downing, DVM. AAHA Press, 2000.

*Smart Medicine for Healthier Living*, by Janet Zand, LAc, OMD, Allan N. Spreen, MD, CNC and James B. LaValle, RPh, ND. Avery Publishing Group, Inc., 1999.

*Sparky Fights Back: A Little Dog's Big Battle Against Cancer*, by Josee Clerens and John Clifton. Foley Square Books, 2005.

*Survive Your Cancer: The Essential Who, What, Where, When & How Guide for Cancer Patients & Their Families*, by Barbara Brandon. Survivor's Wisdom, 2003.

*The Complete Herbal Handbook for the Dog and Cat*, by Juliette De Bairacli Levy. Faber & Faber, 1991.

*The Essential Guide to Natural Pet Care: Cancer*, by Cal Orey. BowTie Press, 1998.

*The Naturally Clean Home: 101 Safe and Easy Herbal Formulas for Non-Toxic Cleansers*, by Karyn Siegel-Maier. Workman Publishing Company, 1999.

*The Nature of Animal Healing: The Definitive Holistic Medicine Guide to Caring for Your Dog and Cat*, by Marty Goldstein, DVM. Ballantine Books, 2000.

*Why is Cancer Killing Our Pets?*, by Deborah Straw. Healing Arts Press, 2000.

## VETERINARY/TEXT/REFERENCE BOOKS

*Canine and Feline Geriatric Oncology: Honoring the Human-Animal Bond,* by Alice Villalobos, DVM, with Laurie Kaplan, MSC, Blackwell Publishing, 2007.

*Manual of Natural Veterinary Medicine: Science and Tradition,* by Susan G. Wynn, DVM and Steve Marsden. Mosby, 2002.

*Small Animal Clinical Oncology,* editors Stephen J. Withrow, DVM, DACVIM (oncology) and E. Gregory MacEwen, VMD, DACVIM (oncology, internal medicine). W.B. Saunders Company, 2001.

*Small Animal Internal Medicine,* by Richard W. Nelson, G. Guillermo Couto etc. al. Mosby, Inc., 1999.

*The Illustrated Veterinary Guide, Second Edition,* by Chris C. Pinney, DVM. McGraw-Hill, 2000.

*Veterinary Oncology Secrets,* by Robert C. Rosenthal, DVM, PhD. Hanley & Belfus, Inc., 2001.

## PRODUCTS

Aloha Medicinals
  (775) 886-6300; [www.dogcancer.net]
AtlasWorldUSA
  (310) 324-6644; [www.agaricusbio.com]
Poly MVA® (AMARC Enterprises, Inc.)
  (800) 960-6760; [www.polymva.com]
Pet Summary
  (706) 247-5743; [www.petsummary.com]
Peaceful Valley Farm Supply
  (888) 784-1722; [www.groworganic.com]
Hug-a-Dog® Harness, D3 Pet Productions
  (800) 444-9475; [www.hug-a-dog.com]
Safety Seat Support Harness™, Four Paws® Products
  (631) 434-1100; [www.fourpaws.com]
Eddie's Wheels™ for Pets
  (888) 211-2700; [www.EddiesWheels.com]

## ORGANIZATIONS

American College of Veterinary Internal Medicine
  (800) 245-9081; [www.acvim.org]
American Animal Hospital Association
  (303) 986-2800; [www.aahanet.or]
Animal Cancer Institute
  [www.animalcancerinstitute.com]
Animal Poison Control Center
  (888) 426-4435; [www.apcc.aspca.org]
Morris Animal Foundation
  (800) 243-2345
  [www.morrisanimalfoundation.org]
The Perseus Foundation
  [www.perseusfoundation.org]
Veterinary Cancer Society
  (619) 474-8929; [www.vetcancersociety.org]

## MEDICAL DISCOUNT/INSURANCE PLANS

Pet's Best Pet Insurance®
  (877) 738-7237; [www.petsbest.com]
  Use discount code 213341

Veterinary Pet Insurance®
  (866) 332-7620; [www.petinsurance.com]
  Use discount code Magic Bullet Fund

Embrace Pet Insurance®
  (800) 511-9172
  [www.embracepetinsurance.com]
  Use discount code 13593881

PetFirst HealthCare®
  (866) 937-7387
  [www.petfirsthealthcare.com]
  Use discount code 99-99-29-6013

# Vaccination Waiver Request

Caretaker's Names _____    Dog's Name  _____

_____    Breed        _____

Telephone _____    Sex  _____

Full Address _____    Color/s  _____

_____    Date of Birth  _____

I certify that I have examined the animal described above. To the best of my knowledge and belief, the statements below are true.

This dog is free from infectious, contagious and/or communicable disease and has been for the past _____ days/months

The dog's caretaker states that the dog has had no known exposure to rabies or any communicable disease during the past ____ days/months

_____ The dog's county of residence is not under a rabies quarantine

_____ The caretaker states that the animal has not bitten anyone within the last 10 days

_____ **I recommend that this animal be exempt from the requirement for rabies vaccination** because of the condition/s noted below. The rabies vaccines, as stated by vaccine manufacturers, are for use <u>in healthy animals only</u>.

_____The animal named above is not considered to be healthy because this animal is currently in treatment for the following medical condition: _____

_____ The animal named above has had an anaphylactic reaction to a prior rabies vaccination and further vaccination could result in serious illness or death.

Veterinarian's Signature _____License # _____Date _____

# EARLY WARNING SIGNS OF CANCER AND ILLNESS IN PETS

## *Give Your Pet an At-Home Check-Up Every Month!*

Every caretaker should be familiar with these early warning signs.
Early detection ensures the best chance of treatment success.

Conduct an at-home check-up on your pet every month. If you detect any of the signs below, inform your veterinarian but DO NOT PANIC! Many of these signs warn of illnesses that are easily treated.

### SIGNS YOU CAN **FEEL**

**Abnormal Swellings** that continue to grow in the skin, including enlarged lymph nodes

**Abnormal Lumps** in the mouth, mammary glands, testicles, abdomen or at vaccine sites

**Sores or Ulcers** that do not heal in 2 weeks on the nose, ear tips and face — seen particularly on white cats and on the white underside of dogs including Italian Grayhounds, Whippets and Bull Dogs

### SIGNS YOU CAN **SEE**

**Sudden or Progressive Weight Loss** Use a baby scale to weigh cats and small dogs

**Pale Gums and Mucous Membranes** Yellow (jaundice) membranes, bruising, slow or inadequate refill

**Bad Breath** Halitosis or more than one loose tooth at same location

**Abdominal Signs** Distended abdomen, fluid in the abdomen

**Skin Signs** Small red spots or red discoloration of the skin, unexplained bleeding at any location, especially from body openings

### SIGNS YOU CAN **OBSERVE**

**Decreased Appetite** Eating less than usual, walking away from bowl, refusing favorite treats

**Reduced Activity** Lethargy, exercise intolerance, lameness, painful movement, painful joints, hesitation to exercise

**Abnormal Urination** Difficulty urinating, blood in the urine, excessive urine output, increased water drinking

**Abnormal Defecation** Loose stools, diarrhea, straining to defecate, constipation, blood or moucus in the stool

**GastroIntestinal Signs** Difficulty eating, excessive salivation, spitting up food, vomiting food or bile

**Respiratory Signs** Chronic sneezing, discharge from the eyes, unilateral nasal discharge, noisy breathing, trouble breathing, coughing, gagging

**Cardiovascular Signs** Weakness, disorientation, dizziness, paralysis, pain, fainting, breathlessness, increased panting, anxiety

ASK YOUR VETERINARIAN TO DEMONSTRATE OR CLARIFY ANY PART OF THE AT-HOME CHECK-UP THAT YOU DON'T COMPLETELY UNDERSTAND

*Exam room poster available to veterinarians on request. (914) 941-0159. By Alice Villalobos, DVM. Edited and designed by Laurie Kaplan/JanGen Press.*

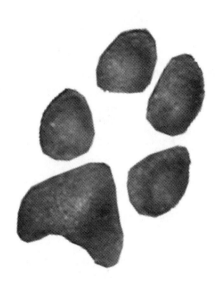

# THE MAGIC BULLET FUND

At this moment, thousands of cancer-dog caretakers are struggling to accept the harsh reality that they will not be able to provide cancer treatment for their adored and adoring canine family members. Those of us who are able to provide treatment for our pups with cancer are very fortunate. Those who cannot afford treatment need your help.

To this end, I established a fund that provides financial assistance to these people, to give their dogs a chance to survive cancer. In honor of my own cancer survivor, the fund is called The Magic Bullet Fund.

The Magic Bullet Fund needs your support. Please meet the dogs currently in treatment. Chat with their caretakers. They need your moral support and compassion. And if you are able to, help us bring some of these beautiful dogs through treatment.

When you purchased this book, I made a contribution to the Fund. Now it's your turn! Please go to The Magic Bullet Fund web site to read about the dogs in treatment. Join the forum, write messages to the dogs' caretakers, ask questions. When you find a pup whose story touches you, donate to help us pay for that dog's treatment.

***JOIN THE MAGIC BULLET FUND FORUM!***
Meet the dogs and their caretakers

http://forums.delphiforums.com/MBFdogs/start

***DONATE ONLINE TO HELP THE MBF DOGS***
www.TheMagicBulletFund.org

***DONATE BY MAIL***
Send check payable to:
The Magic Bullet Fund
PO Box 2574
Briarcliff, NY 10510

**On behalf of all of the dogs
who will have a chance to survive cancer...
On behalf of the people
who love those dogs...**
*Thank you for your generosity!*

*Laurie*

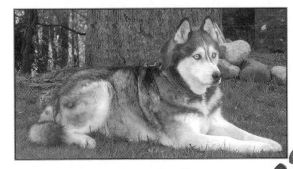

*& Bullet*

Signed copies of this book may be purchased directly from the publisher. If you provide the name of your dog, the author will be happy to inscribe a personal message to you and your dog!

Order online at www.HelpYourDogFightCancer.com

Call (914) 941-0159

Quantity discounts are available to book distributors and resellers. Please contact the publisher by Email at email@jangenpress.com or by telephone above.